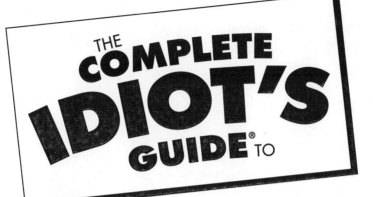

THE COMPLETE IDIOT'S GUIDE® TO

Vegan Eating for Kids

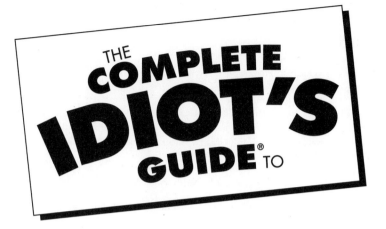

Vegan Eating for Kids

by Dana Villamagna, M.S.J., and Andrew Villamagna, M.D., M.Sc.

ALPHA

A member of Penguin Group (USA) Inc.

ALPHA BOOKS

Published by the Penguin Group

Penguin Group (USA) Inc., 375 Hudson Street, New York, New York 10014, USA

Penguin Group (Canada), 90 Eglinton Avenue East, Suite 700, Toronto, Ontario M4P 2Y3, Canada (a division of Pearson Penguin Canada Inc.)

Penguin Books Ltd., 80 Strand, London WC2R 0RL, England

Penguin Ireland, 25 St. Stephen's Green, Dublin 2, Ireland (a division of Penguin Books Ltd.)

Penguin Group (Australia), 250 Camberwell Road, Camberwell, Victoria 3124, Australia (a division of Pearson Australia Group Pty. Ltd.)

Penguin Books India Pvt. Ltd., 11 Community Centre, Panchsheel Park, New Delhi—110 017, India

Penguin Group (NZ), 67 Apollo Drive, Rosedale, North Shore, Auckland 1311, New Zealand (a division of Pearson New Zealand Ltd.)

Penguin Books (South Africa) (Pty.) Ltd., 24 Sturdee Avenue, Rosebank, Johannesburg 2196, South Africa

Penguin Books Ltd., Registered Offices: 80 Strand, London WC2R 0RL, England

Publisher: *Marie Butler-Knight*
Editorial Director: *Mike Sanders*
Senior Managing Editor: *Billy Fields*
Senior Acquisitions Editor: *Karyn Gerhard*
Senior Development Editor: *Christy Wagner*
Senior Production Editor: *Megan Douglass*
Copy Editor: *Emily Garner*

Cartoonist: *Steve Barr*
Cover Designer: *Becky Batchelor*
Book Designer: *Trina Wurst*
Indexer: *Angie Bess*
Layout: *Ayanna Lacey*
Proofreader: *Laura Caddell*

Contents at a Glance

Contents

Foreword

A vegan meal is a real gift, providing health power that meaty, cheesy meals cannot match. Parents who serve vegan meals do their children an enormous favor, and children who are raised with a vegan menu gain tremendous advantages. Many years ago, researchers learned that vegetarian children reach the same height as nonvegetarian children. And they tend to be slightly leaner, less likely to carry that bit of chubbiness too many other children have these days. Studies also suggest that vegan children have higher IQs than their omnivorous classmates. And on average, they will live years longer. More importantly, when children learn about healthy vegan foods early in life, they are well prepared to avoid the health challenges that adults face.

The American Dietetic Association has reported that not only are plant-based diets acceptable for children; these diets provide real advantages. They report that, "Well-planned vegetarian diets are appropriate for individuals during all stages of the life cycle, including pregnancy, lactation, infancy, childhood, and adolescence, and for athletes …. [A] vegetarian diet is associated with a lower risk of death from ischemic heart disease. Vegetarians also appear to have lower low-density lipoprotein cholesterol levels, lower blood pressure, and lower rates of hypertension and type 2 diabetes than nonvegetarians. Furthermore, vegetarians tend to have a lower body mass index and lower overall cancer rates."

Serving healthful vegan meals is easy. After all, think how simple it is to cook a batch of oatmeal in the morning, or zap some veggie sausage links. How easy it is to pack a sandwich with veggie bologna slices that look and taste just like regular bologna, cook veggie dogs instead of regular hotdogs, or heat up baked beans without that hunk of pork. Whether you're cooking from scratch or using convenience foods, the vegan choices have the edge when it comes to health and are quick and easy enough for even the busiest parents.

Although you will learn much more about healthful nutrition in the pages that follow, let me say a word here about complete nutrition. A healthful menu is drawn from what are sometimes called the New Four Food Groups—vegetables, fruits, whole grains, and legumes. These staples translate into a bowl of hearty breakfast oatmeal or cold cereal with soy milk or rice milk. Lunch might be bean chili, a veggie hot dog with baked beans, or pasta salad with a green salad. Dinner could be a vegetable soup, spaghetti with tomato sauce, and steamed veggies, or one of a thousand other possibilities. These foods provide plenty of protein, even without careful combining (or "complementing") of food groups. Any normal variety of plant foods, consumed over the course of a day, provides the complete protein a growing child needs. You'll find plenty of calcium and iron in green vegetables and beans, as well as in fortified foods, for those who want them.

It is essential to provide a reliable source of vitamin B_{12}, which should generally mean providing a multivitamin daily, although vitamin B_{12} is also found in fortified foods, such as vitamin-fortified soy milk and cereals. I recommend a daily multivitamin for all children, not only vegans.

To all parents who have chosen to provide vegan foods at home, let me say that your children are lucky to have you as their parents. Not every parent yet realizes what a difference it makes. When health authorities first recommended smoke-free environments for children, some parents were a bit slow to take the advice. When child-safety car seats became mandatory, it took some time before their benefits were widely appreciated. Ditto for bicycle helmets and athletic safety gear. But the data are now in, and we now know that taking a bit of extra care of our children can really pay off. Nowhere are the benefits more immediate or more powerful than in the contents of their plates.

Providing vegan meals for children is a huge favor. Your children will thank you, and so do I.

Dr. Neal Barnard
President of the Physicians Committee for Responsible Medicine

Introduction

Raising vegan kids in a world full of cheeseburgers, ice cream, and pizza can seem like an impossibly daunting task. You can sometimes feel like you're fighting a losing battle. But take heart! We're here to tell you that it's not only *possible*, it's *admirable*.

Eating a vegan diet is a healthful choice for ourselves, for our children, and for the planet. According to *Pediatrics in Review*—widely viewed as the gold standard journal in up-to-date kids' health information—"Multiple experts have concluded independently that vegan diets can be followed safely by infants and children without compromise of nutrition or growth and *with some notable health benefits*." (Italics added.)

As adults, it's not always easy to be a food contrarian, and it can be even more challenging for kids. But motivated, resourceful parents can find ways to make anything, including veganism, work to their child's advantage.

Different readers may come to this book for different reasons, but all with the common goal of helping the kids you love be healthy and happy eating vegan all the time, most of the time, or more often than not. How you came to that decision is as unique as your situation.

Perhaps you've been vegan since high school or college. Maybe you've been health conscious about your own vegan diet, or maybe not so much. But now, with a baby on the way or a little one ready to try solid foods, you're ready to step up your nutrition game. Yet, like most new parents, you're not exactly sure how to introduce your child to eating (in this case, vegan style), or exactly what she needs nutritionally to grow and thrive at different stages. You'll find all that in this book.

Did your school-age child announce she doesn't want to eat animal products anymore? Out of love for animals or a desire to help the environment, your child is proclaiming, "No more meat! No more milk! No more eggs!" The media devotes lots of coverage these days to the cruelty of factory farms, the positive work of animal compassion groups, and the environmental impact of animal products and veganism, so it's no surprise kids are taking notice and declaring their change of heart at the dinner table. Find out how to support them, and why you may want to take the plunge, too.

Or maybe your child is becoming vegan by default as one among many in the ever-increasing number of kids with allergies or sensitivities to dairy, eggs, or the additives and hormones in meat.

If your entire family is starting out on the vegan road together, you need to be sure each family member's needs are met. This isn't one-size-fits-all because kids at every stage of growth have unique sets of nutritional and social needs we parents need to tune in to.

Whatever your motivation, now that you're here you'll:

◆ Get the 411 on vitamins and calories

◆ Find out how to talk to your child's doctor about vegan diets

◆ Learn to make vegan pancakes, a delicious vegan birthday cake, and quick vegan snack bags

◆ And more!

With tons of health, nutrition, kitchen, and social tips, and 35 kid-friendly vegan recipes, *The Complete Idiot's Guide to Vegan Eating for Kids* helps you navigate your child's vegan food options and choices. By starting with a few simple nutrition guidelines and safeguards, adding some flexibility, throwing in a heaping spoonful of community and a dash of creativity, you've got the recipe for healthy, fun, vegan family living for you and your kids.

The tide is turning toward plant-based diets. You and your kids can ride the wave to greater health, increased animal compassion, and a better Earth.

How This Book Is Organized

The Complete Idiot's Guide to Vegan Eating for Kids is divided into four parts. We take you from the health, dietary, and social basics to more specific nutritional needs for kids at different ages and stages. Then we cover the nuts and bolts of a kid-friendly vegan kitchen, including 30+ kid-tested, food-writer-mom–created and doctor-dad–approved recipes.

Here's how it all breaks down:

Part 1, "The Basics of Raising a Vegan Child," outlines why being a vegan kid is achievable and healthy, yet sometimes incredibly tricky. We've included lots of motivating news from health studies on the benefits of vegan diets for kids, as well as why it's important to consider taking vegan ideals into your choices for your child's toys, clothes, and more. You'll be encouraged to examine your own family's beliefs and boundaries about what is and isn't "vegan enough." You can debunk the most common myths about vegan kids with comebacks we provide for the next family holiday meal. Finally, you learn how to teach your child to deal with some real-world dilemmas like school lunchroom politics and what to say when grow-ups ask them about their food choices.

Part 2, "Nutritional Needs of Vegan Kids," covers the specifics parents need to know to be sure their vegan child is getting enough of all the essential vitamins and nutrients to grow up healthy and strong without animal-based foods. First up, the needs of vegan babies and toddlers, including how to find a veg-friendly doctor for your child's medical care. Next, discover what vegan kids ages 4 through 8 need to thrive, including special tips for picky eaters. Then, find out what vegan tweens ages 9 through 13 need as they hit the onset of puberty and hormones begin to kick in. In the unlikely event that your child's vegan diet isn't working, Part 2 also includes tips on how to discern the problem and what to do to correct course.

Part 3, "Stocking the Vegan Kitchen," targets those three dreaded parent activities: grocery shopping with kids; fitting a healthful diet into a tight budget; and cooking meals everyone in the family will eat, from youngest to oldest. We talk about what you need to stock the best vegan home kitchen and ways to involve your child in preparing meals and other fun foods together.

Part 4, "Let's Eat!" is, of course, our favorite section. Here's where we get to show you the amazingly easy, kid-tested and -approved recipes we've created through the last 12 years of kitchen fun. A lot of fancy, delicious vegan cookbooks are out there—and we love them all. But many recipes in them cater to vegan singles or couples with ample time and energy to shop at five different specialty stores, come home and cook for two hours, and serve a four-course meal. The recipes in this book cater to real-world parents like us who have little time, even less energy, and multiple hungry little mouths to feed. Most recipes are relatively quick, made with readily available ingredients, and include variations to make them pleasing to both kid and adult palates.

At the back of the book we include a glossary of helpful terms and more kid-focused vegan resources to help you continue on your own family's journey into healthy, yummy, compassionate eating.

Extras

In every chapter, you'll find these boxes of helpful, important, or fun info to make your job feeding vegan kids easier:

> **That's So Vegan**
>
> Check out these boxes for facts about veganism, health notes, and vegan kitchen tips.

> **Parent Trap**
>
> Be sure to read these cautionary notes to help you keep your child safe and healthy.

> **Vegan Vocab**
>
> Here you'll find definitions that help you better understand the technical aspects of child health and nutrition.

> **Vegan Voices**
>
> These boxes contain advice from vegan parents. We've surveyed more than 60 vegan parents from around the globe and brought their top tips to you.

Acknowledgments

We'd like to thank our agent, Marilyn Allen; Senior Acquisitions Editor Karyn Gerhard, Senior Development Editor Christy Wagner, and everyone who assisted with the creation of this book at Alpha Books; Dr. Neal Barnard, for writing the foreword, and the entire PCRM staff for the important work they do; all the vegan parents who graciously

shared their families' experiences; Drew's colleagues who offered information and opinions; *VegNews, Vegetarian Times,* Peta.com, and other
progressive magazines and websites for endless inspiration, motivation
and for being the voice for change; Michelle Crouch, freelance writer
extraordinaire, for the push; our children, for sampling endless recipe
creations (some winners, some flops); Bev and Bob, for always supporting and encouraging their kids and grandkids to do good work
and make the world a better place. And thanks to Garcia, our black
Labrador, the "Other Mother" in our family.

Trademarks

All terms mentioned in this book that are known to be or are suspected
of being trademarks or service marks have been appropriately capital-
ized. Alpha Books and Penguin Group (USA) Inc. cannot attest to the
accuracy of this information. Use of a term in this book should not be
regarded as affecting the validity of any trademark or service mark.

Part 1

The Basics of Raising a Vegan Child

No doubt about it, a well-balanced vegan diet is healthful for children. But there are still many myths surrounding veganism, as well as a lot of positive information that never sees the light of mainstream media. Once you read the facts about the health advantages of a vegan diet for kids and the veg-positive truths hiding behind the negative myths, you will be even more confident about your food choices.

Part 1 covers the basics of raising a vegan child. Find out how you can identify your own family's views on vegan issues, large and small. Explore ways to handle situations unique to vegan kids. And learn even more reasons to be proud of raising a vegan child.

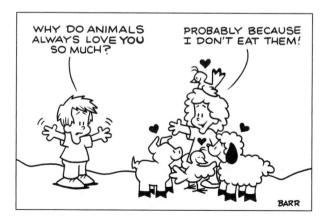

Vegan Advantages for Kids

In This Chapter

- ◆ Health plusses for vegan kids
- ◆ The environmental benefits of being vegan
- ◆ It's about more than just the food

Savvy parents know simply assuming children will grow up strong, slim, and disease-free in today's world full of fast-food, TV commercials, and environmental toxins is much too naive. The $10 billion-a-year, kid-targeted food and beverage marketing industry's goal is to get kids to ask for fast food and junk food. Parents, we need to tell our kids what these marketers are up to and where that "desirable" food actually comes from. We need to provide alternative messages to our kids about what's really good for them. We need to show them how eating healthy—and especially eating vegan—can taste good, or our kids will drift away into a sea of fatty burgers, shakes, and fries with so many other twenty-first century American children.

Even the federal government, which has set a rather sad but seemingly achievable goal of "only" a 5 percent obesity rate among American children, admits we're losing the battle. The most recent federal survey (2003 to 2006) of American children's health showed that about *17 percent* of American children ages 6 to 19 are obese—that's 30 pounds over ideal body weight.

Many families choose a vegan lifestyle for ethical, compassionate, and environmental reasons, no doubt. But if protection against this obesity epidemic and overall improved health for your child isn't one of the driving forces for your choice, don't be surprised if it's one of the side effects.

The Health Benefits of Being Vegan

A plant-based, animal-product-free diet can't quell all health threats, but it can certainly reduce the risk many of them pose to your child's short- and long-term health outlook. Vegan diets have been shown to reduce the incidence of high blood pressure, type 2 diabetes, high cholesterol, certain types of cancer, and obesity-related illnesses.

If you follow a few important but simple guidelines (especially taking care to supply necessary vitamin B_{12}), your child's nutritional needs can easily be met without the inclusion of animal products—all the while setting her on a much wider road to life-long health with fewer pitfalls than her meat-, dairy-, and egg-consuming playmates.

That's So Vegan _____

A recent study by the U.S. Centers for Disease Control places the number of vegetarian kids at 0.5 percent of American youth. Other studies cite the number of vegetarian American kids ages 8 to 18 at about 3 percent. Compare that with stats that show 17 to 30 percent of American youth are overweight to obese, and it's clear we've got a long way to go to get the numbers right.

Kids Are Naturally Healthy, Right?

It's shocking, but true: doctors are now diagnosing children as young as 4 years old with obesity-related diseases such as type 2 diabetes, high blood pressure, fatty liver disease, and musculoskeletal problems. In the past, these problems showed up in 40- to 50-year-olds, not kids.

Who's to blame? Considering that parents are largely who decide what children eat at least through the tween years, when kids have preventable health problems, the responsibility lands squarely on those parents' shoulders. Other adults in children's lives, from caretakers, to school officials, to society at large, also play a role.

The good news is, most of these illnesses can be avoided—or even reversed—through dietary changes, especially a vegan diet. It's up to us parents to stock our fridges and pantries with good nutrition for our children and teach them about healthful eating so they can make the right choices when they're away from home or at school.

Have a Heart

The only thing kids' hearts should be full of is love. But clogged arteries are a reality for far too many American kids. The American Academy of Pediatrics suggested medications to lower the "bad" type of *cholesterol*, LDL (low-density lipoprotein), for thousands of children whose levels are too high.

A🍎C   Vegan Vocab _____

> **Cholesterol** is a fat found in all animal fats and oils. It can be found in every cell of the human body and is used to build healthy cells, as well as some vital hormones. High cholesterol contributes to fatty deposits in blood vessels, which increases the risk of a heart attack or stroke.

Preventing heart disease starts as early as babyhood by breast-feeding. Human breast milk is the only mammalian milk that's tailor-made for human children. According to one study, babies who breast-feed for 1 month or longer have lower body mass index and higher levels of good HDL (high-density lipoprotein) cholesterol in midadulthood than adults who were bottle-fed. Add a vegan diet and regular exercise, and you've got the recipe for a heart-healthy life.

What exactly is it about plant-based diets that protect the heart? Elevated blood cholesterol increases the risk of heart disease. Cholesterol is only manufactured in the human body and in the bodies of animals. Diets based on grains, fruits, vegetables, nuts, and seeds and devoid of animal products predictably do not contribute to high cholesterol. In one study in Britain, cholesterol levels of lacto-ovo vegetarians (vegetarians who consume dairy and egg products) were 14 percent higher than in vegans.

Fiber intake is another pro-player in the anticholesterol game, and vegan diets have tons of fiber. According to the *Journal of the American College of Nutrition*, "vegans generally consume 50 percent to 100 percent more fiber than the general population, and soluble fiber from legumes, fruits, vegetables, nuts, and seeds appears to reduce heart disease risk by lowering plasma cholesterol." Vegans also eat much less saturated fat, another contributor to high cholesterol, than omnivores.

Heart disease is the number-one killer of adults in America. A vegan diet is undoubtedly the heart-healthy choice.

Ever Met an Obese Vegan?

Try really, really hard, and even your vegan child could become obese. After all, cookies, cotton candy, potato chips, and many types of french fries are animal-product-free foods. Most vegans and vegetarians, however, are not overweight. Meat eaters have three times the obesity rate of vegetarians, and *nine times* that of vegans.

According to the Archives of Pediatrics and Adolescent Medicine, American children today are plagued with higher rates of obesity than ever before. Nearly 1 in 5 American 4-year-olds are clinically obese. Beyond obesity-related illnesses, the social stigma and low self-esteem obese children face in school can be almost certainly avoided by a healthy vegan diet and regular playtime exercise.

Cancer Protection

Any parent winces when they hear the words *childhood cancer.* Sadly, 46 American kids are diagnosed with cancer every school day, or more than 2,600 cases each year. That includes childhood leukemia as well as cancers and tumors of the brain, bones, lymph system, muscles, and kidneys.

Some childhood cancers have been associated with nitrites, a preservative used in meat hot dogs. According to the Cancer Prevention Coalition, studies indicate, "children born to mothers who consumed hot dogs one or more times per week during pregnancy have approximately double the risk of developing brain tumors. Children who ate hot dogs one or more times per week were also at higher risk of brain cancer."

And hot dogs aren't the only problematic animal-based food when it comes to cancer. Bad compounds called HCAs (heterocyclic amines) form in beef, pork, chicken, and fish cooked at high temperatures in methods such as barbecuing, grilling, and broiling. National Cancer Institute (NCI) researchers have identified 17 different HCAs that result from cooking muscle meats at high temperatures. According to the NCI, studies have shown an increased risk of developing colorectal, pancreatic, and breast cancers with high intakes of well-done, fried, or barbecued meats.

Diet alone cannot protect against all cancers, and cancer survival rates have risen dramatically in the past 25 years. Still, vegan kids don't eat hot dogs or muscle meats—one less worry for parents, thanks to veganism.

Allergies

Dangerous food allergies and pesky, bad-mood-inducing, stomach-cramping food sensitivities plague many children. In fact, the U.S. Centers for Disease Control estimates 1 in 26 kids battle a food allergy. Over 90 percent of the most severe food allergies in childhood are caused by eight foods:

- Cow's milk
- Fish
- Hen eggs
- Peanuts

- Shellfish
- Soy
- Tree nuts (and seeds)
- Wheat

But vegan kids don't have to worry about dairy (including the more mild but still bothersome lactose intolerance), egg, seafood, or meat allergies.

Puberty Slow-Down

According to information published by the Physicians Committee for Responsible Medicine (PCRM), "diets rich in animal protein, found in meat, eggs, and dairy products, appear to reduce the age of puberty."

PCRM sites a study from the Harvard School of Public Health in 2000, which found that girls who consumed higher levels of animal protein compared to vegetable protein between 3 and 8 years of age began to menstruate earlier. Doctors say that early onset of menses increases women's chances of female cancers. And hey, don't kids grow up too fast these days anyway, without puberty coming early, too?

Illnesses, Pathogens, and Toxins

A top-tier reason not to eat meat or serve it to your children: mad cow disease (or any other food-borne illness associated so often with animal products). Vegans can let their kids lick the beaters from cookie and cake batter without the fear of them ingesting salmonella bacteria, which raw eggs (as well as other poultry) may contain. Soft cheeses may harbor the bacterium listeria, most dangerous for pregnant moms and their unborn babies. Drink raw (unpasteurized) cow's milk—very popular in the nonvegan, health-conscious community—and run the risk of ingesting salmonella, E coli, and listeria. Undercooked pork carries the concern of parasites, and eating large fish now means ingesting mercury, to the extent that the Food and Drug Administration (FDA) warns children and pregnant or lactating women not to eat fish more than twice a week.

Bottom line: vegan kids bypass almost all those animal-product-borne pathogens and problems.

Parent Trap

Unfortunately, food-borne pathogens are not limited to animal products. Outbreaks of E coli on spinach and tomatoes have prompted the FDA to issue a number of widespread food recalls. To protect your child, wash fruits and vegetables thoroughly—which cuts but doesn't eliminate risk (only cooking does that)—and peel foods that make sense to do so. Watch health news for outbreaks and recalls. If an outbreak occurs, avoid the risk altogether until the outbreak ends.

The Best of Everything

Veganism is based on what's quickly becoming common sense in nutrition and disease prevention. The federal government's "Fruits and Veggies—More Matters" campaign (formerly called "5 A Day") encourages all Americans to eat more fruits and vegetables. For kids whose families follow a plant-based diet, that's already a no-brainer.

The Physicians Committee for Responsible Medicine's Cancer Project teaches health-care providers, patients, and kids how to eat delicious, plant-based, antioxidant-rich, high-fiber diets to fight cancer.

Michael Pollan, author of the best-seller *The Omnivore's Dilemma*, wrote the book *In Defense of Food* with this mantra in mind: "Eat food. Not too much. Mostly plants." Does that sound like a mostly vegan diet? Seems that vegan families already practice the healthy habits others are finally coming to accept as truth.

Vegan Is as Vegan Does

In addition to what your child eats, what she wears, where she lives, and what she plays with may also impact her health. For many families, promoting health through a vegan lifestyle extends beyond food into clothing, home cleaning supplies, and toys.

The "vegan" label doesn't always equal "organic," but it often does. Finding and buying products that are animal-product-free and not tested on animals may be worth the extra trouble and price for the reduced chemical exposure. Nixing chemicals used in leather treatment, wool, and other animal products; ensuring that your household cleaners are as natural as possible; and buying toys that haven't been treated with harmful coatings—especially for the babies and toddlers, explorers who love to chew on their toys—can also improve your child's chances of growing up healthy.

The man-made chemical compound known as PCB (polychlorinated biphenyls) has been proven to affect the human endocrine system, especially in unborn babies and children. PCBs manufacturing are now banned, but it can still be found in some old toys and old appliances as well as floating around in our environment via meat, water, and even soil because of its long residual life. Be sure your child washes her hands thoroughly before eating, and try to keep your little one's hands out of her mouth.

A nasty neighbor to PCB is BPA (bisphenol A), used in plastic baby bottles and sippy cups. Use glass or any bottle or cup with a recycling number higher than #5 to be safe.

> **That's So Vegan**
>
> For you iPhone users, the Vegetarian SmartList ($24.99) is an incredible app that catalogues 4,399 foods, drugs, personal care items, cleaning supplies, and more to uncover hidden animal products in these everyday necessities of life.

Edible Ethics

One of the less-tangible, but perhaps no less important, health benefits of vegan eating for kids is the mental health boost that comes from living a life of thoughtful eating. There's a disconnect that kids are required to adapt to as a result of naturally loving animals but also being required to eat them. Kids are told by authority figures in our culture that it's okay to kill and eat some animals but make pets out of others. This kind of confusion in thought and reason is one that may carry over into other aspects of their lives.

Kids tend to naturally be sensitive, honest, and logical. And when they sense disconnects like "we don't eat our dog but you can eat that cow," they're likely to point it out. In his book *The World Peace Diet*, vegan activist Will Tuttle contends that parents who teach their kids it's fine to eat certain animals causes a "forced unawareness," which "becomes a sort of armor, dulling the mind and deadening the vital spiritual spark within us …." On the flip side, supporting your child's natural emotions and logical reasoning is good brain food.

For vegan parents, encouraging kids to listen to and think critically about one of their most basic feelings (love of animals), and how it relates to one of their most basic choices (what they eat), is a gift. Veganism is a healthy way for kids to grow in body, mind, and spirit.

The Least You Need to Know

- A vegan diet can combat some of the most common modern diet-related childhood illnesses, including type 2 diabetes, cancer, and obesity.

- Until kids are teens, parents are the gatekeepers for the kinds of foods that dominate children's lives.

- Beyond food, health-promoting vegan choices include clothing, household cleaners, and toys.

- With the right motivation and education, vegan diets can contribute to a lifetime of better physical, mental, and spiritual health for your child.

Chapter 2

Are You Vegan Enough?

In This Chapter

- What "vegan" means to you
- Talking points for tough stuff
- Be a family on a mission
- If at first you don't succeed, try again

At first glance, the idea of feeding vegan kids seems straight-forward: don't give them any food or drinks made from or by animals. Period.

Then we enter the real world.

Case in point: imagine yourself at a gathering of parents and toddlers where the host has assembled a lovely—but mostly nonvegan—snack table. You are standing near the table talking to a vegan friend and her 3-year-old son. In the midst of your conversation, the little guy steps toward the snack table, paws a carrot stick, and is about to dip it into some obviously nonvegan cheesy dip. Mom lunges at her son, grabbing the erroneously dipped carrot out of his hand, and practically shouts, "Don't eat that!" startling him and everyone else nearby.

This, unfortunately, is a true story—and not the ideal way to handle your child's food faux pas. In this chapter, we take a look at some situations vegans find themselves in and offer some help dealing with them.

What's Vegan Enough?

In an interview on Salon.com, Jeffrey Masson, author of *The Face on Your Plate: The Truth About Food*, describes himself as "veganish" because he occasionally slips up when he's not at home and "accidentally eats, say, a cookie prepared with milk." The article continues: "This vegan's not the sort of purist who would make a scene in public by spitting out an offending morsel."

In an ideal world, most vegan parents would rather their kids eat vegan 100 percent of the time. And in our poll of more than 60 vegan families, about 40 percent said they actually do meet that goal. Another 28 percent of respondents' kids eat vegan more than 90 percent of the time. And for another 20 percent, more than 75 percent of their diet is reportedly vegan in a typical week.

Whatever ideal we set for ourselves and for our children, we can help them be healthy, provide compassionate food choices, and still not become neurotic about food. Vegan or omnivorous, stressful food environments can contribute to eating disorders in families, which is never desirable. Raising vegan kids does not require yelling, grabbing, or stress.

Making the Best of the Situation

Raising vegan children in a world that remains largely carnivorous is still a challenge, if not quite as hostile as it once was. When it comes to kids and their constantly changing stages, tastes, moods, and mistakes, veganism need not be seen as an all-or-nothing, win-or-lose proposition. There's room for error, for taking two steps forward and one step back, for making the best possible choice from the options at hand. In our family, we call this the *BPO*—the *best possible option*.

Vegan Vocab

When you have to make a less-than-perfect food decision for your child because of social circumstance, time pressure, or lack of preferred veg choice, you may have to go with the **BPO**, the **best possible option**. No guilt or shame here. Then reassess what you could do next time to be better prepared with a vegan option.

Especially at first, aim for patterns, not perfection. Look at the grand scheme of your child's overall diet. Don't analyze every morsel he puts in his mouth. The kinder you can be with yourself and your child, the more likely you both will continue to progress and enjoy the vegan way of life.

Consider this example: you and your 4-year-old child are playing in the park with relatively new friends. You're both invited to come back to the friend's house for a casual lunch. Your child has already eaten the vegan snack bag you packed (see Chapter 15). Snack bag consumed, when he's ready for lunch, you don't have an alternative on hand. Upon arrival, the friend's mom offers the kids ham sandwiches, cheese cubes, soda crackers, and grapes on a tray with chocolate milk. You thank the mom, decline the sandwich, offer the grapes and crackers to your child, and ask for water or juice instead of milk. If your child snags a piece of cheese, you may or may not suggest he put it down, depending on the appropriateness of that action in the moment.

You mention casually to the friend that the grapes and crackers are perfect, thank you, and you and your child are vegan. Your child gets to eat, no one is offended, and you've given your friend a tip to keep the cheese in the fridge next time your child comes to play. Then you serve him a sandwich when you get home. That's the BPO.

Creating incremental change in your child's diet comes naturally by first and foremost setting an example with your own. Make vegan eating easy and enticing for your child by providing yummy vegan favorite foods at home. Be true to your child's current stage of development and social needs by being as prepared and as nonconfrontational as possible. In a pinch, keep the BPO in mind.

Media Pressure

Inevitably, your child is going to hear mixed (or just plain wrong) messages about veganism in the media. When they watch or read a story about someone who's vegan, the adjectives *strict* or *militant* will often be attached. The media often portrays vegans as uptight, angry, judgmental, animal-rights-obsessed college kids or punk anarchists who don't yet understand the "real world." On the flip side, the media sometimes likes to glamorize the perfectly vegan movie star, singer, or athlete blessed with a personal chef, 100-acre organic farm, and 25 adopted rescue dogs.

Does your family resemble any of these vegan stereotypes, negative or positive? It's important to counter images of perfection with realistic views of what real-life vegan family living means to your family.

It's also important to arm your kids with correct information for when the naysayers descend, which they will. Casual discussions about veganism sometimes deteriorate into armchair quarterbacks playing the hypocrisy card, pointing out the inconsistencies of vegans who are just doing their level best to live more consciously in a nonvegan world: What if you wear leather? Or take medications derived from animals? Aren't you killing plants to eat them? Crops grown in organic fertilizers aren't really vegan, are they? Plastics, which are derived from oil, which is derived from dinosaurs, aren't technically vegan, are they?

This line of questioning can be exhausting for adult vegans and confusing for kids who haven't been given fair warning that it's bound to happen.

The Debate Continues

Even within the veg community, the "us versus them" debates continue. Angry letters to editors of vegan magazines challenge purist arguments with the question: *am I not vegan enough for you?* The debate about whether honey is acceptable in a vegan diet also continues. (Some say excluding insect products like honey from the vegan diet trivializes the arguments about animal suffering; others believe including any animal product at all clouds the definition.)

No doubt, a lot of the options mentioned in this chapter will rile more than one or two people, as does even just the mention of the term *vegan enough.* For some, that's like saying someone is kind of pregnant. Either you are, or you aren't. That's a debate for another book.

While it's an important debate in the vegan movement at large, this approach may be counterproductive for most kids because kids need more leeway, time, and exceptions to purist rules than adults do. If you stay flexible, creative, and positive, there's a much better chance your child will enjoy vegan eating and make it her own, not just what her family does.

More and more veg-positive media aimed at kids is coming online all the time, as well as in books, in movies, and in other sources. (You'll find many listed in Appendix B.) Talking to people about why you like being vegan or sharing delicious food in your child's classroom or at his birthday party is also a useful way to show the benefits of a vegan family lifestyle. The positive ways to spread the vegan message often use fewer debating words and more delicious food— and are much more effective in the end.

> **That's So Vegan**
>
> One of the best veg-positive media resources for kids currently available is Petakids.com. The "What to Eat" section is particularly useful to veg kids.

Defining Your Own Success

In her book *Get It Ripe,* author and nutritionist jae steele talks about making informed choices and choosing the best option in the moment. We like what she writes here: "One of the worst things you can do is beat yourself up for eating 'bad' food; a close second is policing others for their food choices, and sometimes the two go hand in hand." (steele posts great recipes—many of which are kid-friendly and easy to make— on her blog, domesticaffair.blogspot.com.)

Family Talking Points

When talking to your child about being vegan, especially when he has questions about why he can't eat a certain food his friends eat, be prepared to listen. His struggles as a vegan, especially at school, may be very different from your daily experiences as an adult vegan. Some of the social concerns you won't be able to "fix," but you can show him that you're listening, that you care, and that the world isn't always a fair place, especially for people who are going against the status quo to try to make a change for the better.

Depending on your child's age, he also might ask you a lot of tough questions specifically about veganism and animal products that don't have black-and-white answers. How you answer those questions will differ depending on his maturity level and your comfort with exposing your child to some of the harsher realities of the world of raising animals for food.

> **That's So Vegan**
>
> Find a fun, kid-friendly, and comprehensive education guide about farm animals at www.farmsanctuary.org/education. The three free guides come in levels for elementary school-age, tween, and teen kids. The nonprofit Farm Sanctuary's centers are based in Watkins Glen, New York, and northern California. Consider visiting for a memorable vegan family field trip.

Here are some of the more common kid questions, and some possible responses you can give:

Why do people ask me if I want a hamburger when they know I don't eat meat? I think those people may be uncomfortable with considering the change for themselves, so they make a joke out of it. Or maybe they want to see if you're really committed to not eating meat, so they're testing you. How does it make you feel when they say that to you? How do you respond? Do you like the way you respond?

Why can't we let all the farm animals go (or all the lobsters in the tank at the grocery store, or all the animals in testing facilities, etc.)? I wish we could help those animals be free to live in their natural habitat. But animals on farms and in stores are considered their owner's property. For now, that's the law. What are some other ways we could help animals in those situations?

My teacher says killing a farm animal isn't the same as killing a dog. She says it's slaughtering—not killing—when a farm animal dies for meat. Is that true? Unfortunately, a lot of people do think it's different and it's okay to kill farm animals. Our family disagrees with that. We know farm animals feel emotions like fear, they enjoy lying in the sun, and they connect with their babies, just like dogs. We don't want to intentionally cause any animal harm if we can help it.

Aunt Sally says I won't be strong if I don't eat meat. Is that true? No, that's not true. I want you to grow strong and healthy, and not eating meat can help you do that. Healthy foods like *[list some of his favorites]* will help you grow strong.

Many of these questions are obviously prompted by challenges made to your child's diet by other people such as friends, teachers, and relatives. It's important to let your child know you think he's both capable of and has every right to speak his mind clearly and politely to adults who question his vegan diet.

In the classic parenting book *How to Talk So Kids Will Listen and Listen So Kids Will Talk*, Adele Faber and Elaine Mazlish encourage parents to listen to their kids' feelings about problems but not to be quick to offer advice unless asked. Don't try to shield your child from the realities of being vegan in a nonvegan society (unless repeated bullying has occurred—more on that in Chapter 4). Instead, help kids help themselves by listening, offering to brainstorm options with them for what to say and do when challenged, and trusting that your child will handle the situation well.

Challenging interactions with adults and peers about veganism provide excellent teaching moments for vegan kids. Through this early exposure to the art of standing up for what they believe in, they will learn to stand up for themselves against peer pressure in other instances where the crowd wants them to do something they don't think is right.

That's So Vegan

More than 43 percent of vegan kids in our survey have encountered negative questions or comments about veganism from classmates and friends. And almost 25 percent of families in our survey have experienced the same from at least one of their child's teachers.

Democracy or Dictatorship?

If your child, especially an older tween, follows a vegan or vegetarian diet just because his parents say so—without opportunities for questions, debates, and experimentation—the chances he'll remain vegan into adulthood are likely reduced. Many older kids develop a rebellious streak against anything that is forced upon them.

A child who is allowed some flexibility to experiment with his food choices becomes more self-aware. He learns to tune in to how different foods affect his body, mind, spirit, and social conscience. As you consistently offer healthy, tasty, vegan foods, his palate will almost certainly develop in ways that seek out those comfort foods of home no matter what he experiments with—even perhaps meat—in his teen years. As he learns (predominantly through his parents' example) about vegan diets and has the opportunity to discuss where animal-based foods come from and how they're raised and manufactured, his self-awareness will grow into "other-awareness"—better known as compassion.

Your Child's Food Personality

Depending on your child's unique food personality, he may or may not make eating vegan a piece of cake.

Does your child …

- Like a wide variety of fruits and vegetables?
- Eat veggies both raw and cooked, including salad?
- Try new foods willingly?
- Enjoy exploring ethnic and spicy foods?
- Snack throughout the day?
- Like tofu, seitan, and tempeh cooked in many ways?
- Drink soy, rice, and nut milks?
- Eat handfuls of nuts, seeds, olives, and dried fruits?
- Have a natural aversion to overly sweetened candies and other "fake" foods?

If so, then he's probably an easy vegan.

Does your child …

- Consider apples, bananas, and grapes the only acceptable fruits?
- Eat carrots and celery (or other very common vegetables)—but only slathered with dip?
- Shy away from any other raw vegetable?
- Stick to a basic, same-every-week diet?
- Fear all spicy foods?
- Eat tofu only one way: with barbecue sauce?
- Dislike nondairy milks?
- Have a sweet tooth?

If so, then he's likely a vegan-in-training.

Does your child …

- Consider packaged chewy fruit snacks actual fruit?
- Immediately refuse anything labeled a vegetable?
- Test new foods by placing a tiny bit of the suspicious substance on a utensil and sticking out his tongue to touch it ever so slightly, only to announce he's "tried it" and doesn't like it?
- Like meat?
- Crave sweets, including heavy dairy like ice cream and cheese-cake?
- Live on a diet of food choices you can count on two hands, including peanut butter and jelly (counts as two)?

If so, then you're probably dealing with a reluctant vegan.

No matter what your child's food personality, he can be encour-aged to eat healthier, more compassionately, and yes, vegan. Depending on his age, this will be more or less complicated. "The Picky Eater" section of Chapter 3 is chock-full of tips to motivate your reluctant vegan to branch out and try new, healthier, more compassionate foods. Keep trying. With patience, compromise, and a few tricks and treats, it can be done.

Parent Trap

If your child's food choices are very narrow, or if he eats mainly carbohydrates, tell your doctor. He may need to be evaluated for selective eating disorder, which is linked to sensory disorders. Picky eating may be outgrown, or your child may need some professional help to overcome it and expand his diet to include a healthier range of foods.

Creating a Vegan Family Mission Statement

One very concrete way to define your family's own vegan success is to create a *family mission statement* related specifically to veganism. This means spelling out, in writing, why you want to be a vegan family and what "being vegan" means to your family. Here are some questions you may want to ask about your brand of veganism:

♦ Does it extend beyond food to clothing?

♦ Does it extend beyond human family members to pets?

♦ Does it mean eating vegan at home, and mostly vegan out in the nonvegan world of school, friends, work, and travel?

♦ Do you draw the line at some dairy, no eggs? No eggs, some dairy?

Vegan Vocab

A family mission statement is a shared vision of a family's values, plans, and goals as they relate to the current and future functioning of the family (in this case, as they relate to veganism).

♦ What if a product has no animal products in the ingredients, but says, "may contain traces of milk," due to the manufacturing process? Is that still a vegan option in your family?

♦ What about honey?

♦ Do you allow eggs from chickens raised only by you or friends in conditions you're certain of (as is in the case of Whole Foods founder John Mackey who considers himself vegan but eats eggs from his own free-range chickens)?

♦ Does "being vegan" mean animal-product-free all the time for the adults and mostly vegan most of the time for kids? Or does vegan mean all vegan, all the time for everyone?

♦ What exceptions, if any, will your family make? Birthday parties? Grandma's pie? Not offending your hosts' cultural food norms when traveling to a foreign country?

What are your bottom-line behaviors, so to speak? No meat whatsoever would be one most vegan families can agree upon. Another one might be if there's a vegan option in a situation, it's expected that's the one you'll always choose.

Think about exceptions to rules. What if one of your family members (say, a tween-age son) wants to try to eat meat for a while? Do you allow him to experiment? Does he have to pay for it with his own money, keep it in a separate place in your refrigerator, and prepare it in a different pan bought by him for that purpose? What if one of your children wants to be vegan, other than for Ben and Jerry's Phish Food ice cream? Do you allow one favorite nonvegan product in the home for the reluctant vegan family member?

Whatever the final mission statement looks like, be sure to get input from all family members who are old enough to participate. Even kids as young as preschool age can contribute their thoughts and opinions. The older the child, the more input (and perhaps spirited debates) you'll find coming your way.

Remember, the process of creating the mission statement is as important as the final product. This is the forum for everyone in your family to talk about why they want to be vegan—their thoughts, feelings, fears, reservations, and inspirations—and what they don't want to give up or give in on. Good stuff. Bad stuff. Questions. Beliefs. Ground rules.

Be open to revisit your family statement in 6 months or perhaps every year. Like your family, your idea of "vegan" will likely mature as time goes on. Keep your mind—and your family's dialogue—open.

Off-the-Wagon Moments

There are times—whether it be a meal, a day, a week staying with the grandparents, or even a month or two—when living vegan may be more difficult for your child. This could be due to travel, your work schedule, illness, or just simple daily chaos ramping up a notch or two. All of a sudden your typical vegan lifestyle becomes temporarily derailed.

Don't beat yourself up if your family falls off the vegan wagon. Just take a breath, figure out what you need to change, and hop back on.

If your goal is to be a 100 percent vegan family, rejoice on those days when you and your child's diet hit 100 percent vegan. The days when he's at 90 percent, be thankful he's still eating healthier and more compassionately than most. When it's a 75 percent day, you may want to look for ways to avoid those particular BPO-inducing situations next time. The most important element is staying on your family's path, being enthusiastic about where it leads, and becoming more compassionate to every living being, including yourself and your child.

Of course, every family has to set their own outer limits of what they can and cannot accept. That's where the mission statement and the talking points come in handy. Continue to seek and find a positive balance for yourself, your child, and your family so vegan eating is a gift, rather than a chore. You define your own success.

The Least You Need to Know

- Being a vegan family doesn't have to mean becoming neurotic about food. Stay positive, flexible, and forgiving with your child's food choices.

- Go to the BPO—best possible option—when in a situation where 100 percent vegan choices aren't available.

- Create a vegan family mission statement to help everyone discuss, agree upon, and clarify your individual brand of veganism.

- If your family or your child leaves veganism behind for a time, it's never too late to get back on track.

3

Dealing With Real-World Dilemmas

In This Chapter

- ◆ Problems with picky eaters

- ◆ Sticky family and friend situations

- ◆ Nonvegan authority figures: doctors, childcare providers, and teachers

Beyond home sweet home, there's a big, burly, carnivorous world you and your children must operate within every day. A lot of myths about veganism float around our society largely unchecked (see Chapter 4 for more info on that). It's important to know how to talk to other people in your child's life about her diet, especially when these people may not know much about veganism. Some will be curious, others worried, while others may unfortunately be downright hostile.

In this chapter, we give you tips for how you and your child can talk confidently about vegan eating with everyone from non-vegan extended family to new neighbors. Learn how to open the lines of communication with daycare providers, teachers, and doctors—especially doctors. Because the nonvegan physician/vegan parent relationship can be touchy (depending on how informed your doctor is about vegan diets), we offer a doctor-approved prescription that will help prevent any misunderstandings between you and your child's physician.

Social situations can present dilemmas for vegan parents and kids as well, but after reading this chapter, you and your child will have what it takes to handle them gracefully. But first, let's tackle the trickiest issue of all for vegan parents, one that's closer to home ... in fact, in your home: the picky eater.

The Picky Eater

Even if your child is on board in theory, if she falls into the picky eater category, it may be a challenge to be sure she eats the variety of foods she needs for both proper calorie intake and all essential nutrients (whether she's vegan or omnivorous). In this section, we offer help for turning your picky eater into the next Discovery Channel roving exotic food taster. Okay, maybe you can't coax her into becoming quite *that* adventurous, but this information will provide maximum nutrient benefit from minimum adaptations to her diet, which is sometimes your best bet with picky kids.

If you're raising a picky eater, being a vegan family (and a patient parent) becomes exponentially more difficult. It may be a toddler going through an "eat as little as I can possibly get away with" phase. Or a first-grader who has decided that all food she eats must be warm—not hot, and definitely not cold—nor will she even consider eating anything that has crusts, peels, or seeds. Your picky eater may be a tween who "doesn't like eating dinner anymore" and eats peanut butter and jelly for breakfast and lunch every day for 2 weeks before she gets sick of that food and switches to grilled vegan cheese sandwiches for the following 2 weeks.

Vegan Voices

Keep trying foods. My daughter didn't enjoy avocado or bananas as a baby, but now that she's three they're among her favorite foods.

—Jessica, New York

This, too, shall pass. Meanwhile, it's worth the effort to encourage your picky eater to expand her food horizons a bit and meet her nutritional needs by practicing the three C's: *choice, control,* and *creativity.*

Choice

Offering your child many choices increases the chance she'll find more foods she likes to eat. If your child really balks at eating what you're serving everyone else in the family at dinner, offer her the choice of one or two sides that are simple, nutritious, and easy to make. If she's old enough, encourage her to make one of them herself to share with the family.

Control

Put the greatest possible amount of control over your picky eater's diet in her own hands to avoid further heel-digging. For example, take her grocery shopping to the most well-stocked health food or veg-friendly grocery store in your area and let her pick out five new vegan foods she agrees to try this week. Or if she's truly not hungry at certain times of day like breakfast or dinner, encourage her to eat a snack-size meal at that time but give her the freedom to eat as much healthy food as she wants when she does feel hungry.

Many kids, even picky eaters, will virtually gorge on food when they get home from school. Be sure lots of healthy options are on hand—stock at least one or two that contain a good balance of the major nutrient groups, like protein, fats, and carbs—and give her the control to feel her hunger and satisfy it.

If it's a toddler who seems to be living on air lately, be assured that these little explorers sometimes go through phases where they're too busy learning about the world to slow down and eat much. Focus on high-calorie, high-nutrient drinks like fruit and soy yogurt smoothies and the favorite foods she will eat, watch her bladder and bowel output, and see her doctor for a weight check if the nearly-no-food fast lasts more than a couple weeks or if you're otherwise concerned.

Creativity

Celebrate the power of this final C to get your picky eater out of her food funk. Bring her into the kitchen to choose a recipe that appeals to her and help her create a culinary masterpiece. For younger kids who are still impressed by fun finger food, cut sandwiches, fruits, and veggies into fun shapes like hearts, stars, and triangles.

> **That's So Vegan**
>
> The Vegan Lunchbox blog (www.veganlunchbox.blogspot.com) continually delights with amazingly creative lunchbox creations that may impress your child so much she'll forget about being picky at school lunchtime or at home.

If your tween likes books, take her on a trip to the nearest bookstore and let her pick out one or two fun, beautiful, new cookbooks that interest her. After she has a chance to look them over, head to the grocery store for a tween-led shopping expedition. Then, help her prepare the recipes she's selected. She may eat better than you've ever witnessed when choices and control are combined with the most powerful C of all: creativity.

Finally, unless your child has a more serious eating challenge (see Chapter 2 and Chapter 8 for signs of eating disorders) most picky eaters will favor at least one reasonably healthy standby in each basic nutrient category: protein, complex carbohydrate, fat. If that's veggie nuggets, be sure to always have some in the fridge to include with her dinner when what you've made for the family is unacceptable to her picky palate. If your child likes whole-wheat bread but doesn't want to put anything on it, make or buy the most nutrient-packed bread. If she'll eat nut butters directly from a spoon but not on the bread, give her the spoon and let her eat the bread plain.

In a few years, when she's calling from college to tell you about the fantastic hummus sandwich with sprouts, avocado, and roasted red pepper spread she just ate at the hip coffee shop where she studies (and asking, "Why didn't you ever cook cool stuff like that for me, Mom?"), you'll look back and laugh at the hoops you had to jump through to be sure your child grew up healthy—and be glad you did.

That's So Vegan _____

The ace in the hole for dealing with a picky eater? Vitamins. We talk more in Part 2 about choosing the best vegan vitamins for kids at different stages and needs, but until then, remember: if your child is a picky eater, a vitamin supplement beyond B is necessary for optimal health and growth—at least until her food choices expand.

Mom's Vegan, Dad's Not

You should never discuss religion and politics at a dinner party, right? You may be able to avoid those hot-button topics at a party, but it's almost impossible not to discuss them with your mate, and even more difficult not to discuss food. Religion, politics, and food are three of the most combustible topics in life. So it stands to reason they're in partnerships, too. If mixed-religion or two-party couples can navigate Christmas and Hanukkah, or Republicans and Democrats, then vegan-nonvegan parents can surely figure out how to raise their child amid dietary and philosophical differences, too.

When one parent is vegan and the other isn't, it's imperative that both adults discuss what this means for your child's diet. Otherwise, feelings will get hurt, people will get angry, and the child will be stuck in the middle. In this situation, the family mission statement mentioned in Chapter 2 becomes even more important. Your partner's current position on food ethics and preferences should be heard (understanding that they may evolve), yours voiced as well, compromises made, and boundaries set. This will be easier if the nonvegan parent is vegetarian and more difficult if one is carnivorous.

As in all parenting situations, what's best for the child must take precedence. If you're in a divorce situation, a discussion with a family therapist regarding how to come to an agreement about your child's diet may be warranted.

Vegan Voices _____

Each night, I fix a vegan meal and my husband fixes whatever meat he wants to eat, and our children make food choices. So far it seems to be working out for us!

—Sheri, Wisconsin

If you're the vegan parent in this equation, be prepared to bend a little. If the other parent has emotional attachments to, say, a tradition of buying your child a chocolate ice-cream cone at the neighborhood pool's concession stand after a swim, then a soy ice-cream cone at home isn't likely going to cut it. Yes, we've always been told it's unhealthy to equate food with love, but in reality it often happens. In instances like that, the BPO (best possible option—see Chapter 2) may be to give a little on one or two sentimental choices, draw the line at the most egregious requests (cancer-causing hot dogs at baseball games, for example), and ask the pool concession manager to start selling soy or rice milk–based frozen treats.

Parent Trap

In *Talking to Tweens: Getting It Right* Before *It Gets Rocky with Your 8- to 12-Year-Old*, parenting expert Elizabeth Hartley-Brewer lists "arguments between parents—and feeling marooned in between them" as one of the situations kids are most likely to find stressful. Sometimes agreeing to disagree about veganism with a nonvegan partner and coming to a compromise for your child's diet is best for everyone.

And who knows? If you, the vegan parent, continue to set a stellar example of how happy, healthy, and calm veganism makes you, your partner may just come around sooner than you think. (And it never hurts to keep a fabulous vegan dessert in the house at all times as a positive temptation to nudge them over to the vegan side of life!)

The Cool Friend Isn't Vegan

Many vegan children are so proud they can care for animals by being vegan it simply doesn't matter what their friends are eating. But every now and again, especially when your child enters the tween years, you may come across "the cool friend." You know, the one whose family does everything right and better than yours—including pepperoni pizzas; rib roasts; and sleepover breakfasts of sausage links, bacon, eggs, and French toast.

Watch for the P-word to come into play for your tween. Being vegan may or may not be the "in" thing with the popular crowd at your child's school or homeschool group (although take heart, it's getting cooler all the time). If it's not, she may become embarrassed about what she was once so certain of. This is not only unsettling to her, but often it can be a little more than discouraging to you, the parent. When this happens, it's time to talk.

In *Talking to Tweens: Getting It Right* Before *It Gets Rocky with Your 8- to 12-Year-Old*, Elizabeth Hartley-Brewer emphasizes how important friends are to a tween's blossoming self. Sure, they still rely on us to get most of their security and sense of belonging (even though it may not seem like it sometimes), but they have to be able to try on new ways of being, too, to strengthen their own identity.

"Different friends like to do different things, and these additional activities can be sampled, alongside different cultures, *food and ways of living* [italics added] as they visit different homes," writes Brewer.

Depending on the strength of your child's opinion on the matter, you might want to consider allowing your tween to choose whether she wants to sample her friend's food choices when at the cool family's home. Or you may choose to instruct your child in the fine art of declining politely. Maybe even prepare a yummy vegan dessert with your child to take to the friend's house.

Most importantly, talk to your child and find out her thoughts and feelings. This will help clarify the right course of action to take. And remember, your child isn't the only one who gets to share her feelings. Express your feelings about what's going on with her, too, just per-haps in a more moderated, adult way. Don't judge or dictate; just share feelings. Keep the dialogue flowing, and help your tween check her motivation. Let her know there's a balance between trying new things and caving to peer pressure because she doesn't want to be perceived as "different."

Reasons to Be a Proud Vegan Kid

We're all different, and there are many reasons to be proud of the vegan difference. Here are some talking points your tween can use to express her pride in being vegan:

I'm kind to animals: I don't eat them. Every day, more than 30 million birds and mammals and 45 million fish are killed for food—but not for me! 10 billion animals per year are confined on farms.

I'm saving the environment. I save an acre of trees from being deforested every year by being veg. Food production for a veg diet takes 300 gallons of water, while a meat-eater's diet requires more than 4,000 gallons per day to produce!

I'm not clogging my heart with cholesterol and fat. Twenty-five percent of American kids ages 5 to 10 have elevated cholesterol. 90 percent of kids' diets contain more fat than the recommended level.

I don't just run with the herd. I think for myself about what I eat!

Ways Kids Can Show They're Proud to Be Vegan

To help encourage your child's pride in her vegan lifestyle, here are some fun ways you can support her:

- Buy her a cool veg-message T-shirt or bag from Petacatalog.org.
- Offer a great vegan snack she can take to class.
- Visit a farm sanctuary, and help your child give a class report on it.
- Volunteer together at an animal shelter.
- Help her write a letter to the editor of your newspaper or a kids' magazine about why you're vegan.
- Help her get politically involved by writing letters to politicians about law changes (like Proposition 2 on pig crating in California) or other animal issues.
- Let her choose a veg-positive bumper sticker for the family car (or her bike, guitar case, locker, etc.).

Grandma Knows Best

Okay, this is where things can get really messy, if handled poorly. If one or more of your parents or extended family either frowns upon, complains about, makes fun of, or completely disregards your choice to be a vegan family, how do you stick to your beliefs and keep the intergenerational peace?

Again, the theme of food = love comes into play here, and if the only way Grandma knows to show her food love to her grandkids is through meatballs, meatloaf, scrambled eggs, and cheesecake, you may run into some major static.

As soon as this problem arises, take the opportunity to sit down with the concerned grandparent or other close relative and set some boundaries. Back a decade or two, when veganism was still considered outlandish by most people, there were reports of relatives calling child protection authorities on parents for not feeding their kids meat. These days, cooler heads almost always prevail, but you still don't want to unnecessarily fan the flames of anyone's antivegan mind-set.

> **Parent Trap**
>
> In our survey of more than 60 vegan parents, a whopping 77 percent have received negative comments from extended family about their child's diet.

If you have a relative or friend who works in the meat, dairy, food service, or other industry that's involved in manufacturing, selling, or serving animal products, it's wise to have an extra dose of sensitivity. When discussions about you and your child's veganism arise, these folks may feel your choice is a personal attack on their livelihood. Agree to disagree. Straining a relationship with a relative or close friend over personal choices rarely helps anyone come to a better understanding, and it may be detrimental, especially if your child is emotionally attached to this person.

Consider listening to the relative's feelings first before responding. Perhaps find a point of compromise; for instance, allowing your child to eat Aunt Sally's famous pumpkin pie (which contains eggs) at Thanksgiving if she wants to. After listening and perhaps making a compromise, say something like:

> I know you're concerned about the fact that we don't feed meat or other animal products to our daughter. You know we love our child deeply, and we wouldn't take what she eats or her health lightly. We know you love her, too, and she loves you. You're

going to have to trust that we're doing what's best for her and for our family. If you want more information about why vegan diets are healthy for kids, we can provide that for you. But we don't want any further discussion, negative comments, or sideways remarks about this, and we need you to respect that.

Hopefully, that will take care of it. If not, more action on your part may be necessary. You may need to arrive at family functions after the meal portion has ended, or bring all your own food in a cooler with you when you visit for holiday meals. Bring enough of one particularly omnivore-pleasing vegan dish for everyone. Who knows? If your cooking is good enough, Grandma may be convinced to try eating animal-free more often to lower her cholesterol—or at least give you a compliment on your vegan chocolate cheesecake!

Vegan Voices

We don't want our kids to grow up hateful of meat-eaters or with misconceptions or lies about foods, like meat is poisonous. We want to be very honest with them and encourage them to discover the truth for themselves and to make their own decisions. But of course we also want them to be healthy and to have compassion for animals and care for the earth.

—Chandelle, California

In a New Neighborhood

So you moved into the new neighborhood and the first invitation on your door is to the upcoming annual block party … featuring the traditional pig roast. Yes, indeed, a complete pig will be roasting on your very own street next week, and your new friends and neighbors are thrilled to have the new family attend. Just bring a dish to pass and make a small contribution to the pig purchase of $5 a person. What to do?

When your family is the new kid on the block, you may want to tread lightly, but you don't have to pretend to be someone you're not. Depending on what part of the country you've moved into, or even what neighborhood within a city, veganism may be lauded or laughed at. Either way, attend neighborhood gatherings like block parties and bring a vegan dish to pass, but don't necessarily make food ethics part of your introductions right along with where you moved from, what type of work you do, and how old your kids are. It may be rather alienating to stage an anti–pig roast protest within the first month you arrive. (A few years down the road, when you're a well-loved, well-established fixture in the neighborhood, perhaps then you can offer alternatives.)

You don't have to be "That New Vegan Family" (unless you're a family who likes to be contrarian and your kids enjoy it, too). It may be easier to assimilate if everyone finds out more about you before they find out about what you don't eat. If you're confident enough in your vegan cooking skills, be sure to make a casserole or dessert for the family with the new baby on the block or a soup for someone who's sick. Approach it with a positive, connecting attitude, and veganism and neighborliness can go hand-in-hand.

The Concerned Physician

Your relationship with your child's physician is one of the most important you have to cultivate outside of your immediate family. The time to build a respectful, open relationship with your pediatrician or family medicine physician is when your child is healthy and everything's going well. Then, if your child does become ill or has another health or behavioral problem, your physician is more likely to trust your assessments and partner with you on your child's care. The last thing you want as a parent is to consider your child's health-care provider an adversary rather than an advocate.

Sometimes vegan parents are cautioned not to tell their child's physician they feed her a vegan diet. We strongly disagree. Any information about your child's daily habits is important information for your physician to know to most effectively help her stay healthy. Omissions between parents and physicians create suspicion and, even worse, can lead to medical errors and misdiagnoses.

That's So Vegan

Only 33 percent of vegan parents in our survey said they have received negative comments from health-care professionals about their child's vegan diet. Times they are a'changing!

Ideally, you'll find a physician for your child who is personable, competent, and well educated about vegan diets (see Chapter 5 for tips on how to interview a potential doctor). Unfortunately, many doctors know a lot about nutrient deficiencies, obesity-related disorders, and other negatives related to diet, but not much about the specifics of the healthiest diets.

Be prepared to find a physician who may not know much about veganism but whose medical competency you respect, who listens, and who has good rapport with you and your child. Then, in a spirit of partnership, not preaching, educate them about vegan diets for children.

The following is a script on how to talk to a new physician about your child's vegan diet:

> You should know that our family, including "Janie," eats a plant-based, vegan diet. We've done a lot of reading on the subject and feel it's the healthiest way for our family to eat. If you would like, I can provide you with copies of the studies and names of the books I've read.

> We're aware of the vitamin B_{12} concern for people who do not eat animal products, so she takes a daily multivitamin. I've brought the vitamin bottle with us, if you'd like to see what nutrients this particular vitamin includes. I'd be interested in your assessment of the vitamin.

> It's really important to me to partner with you on my daughter's health care, so if you have any questions or concerns about her diet, please feel free to ask. Eating vegan works great for us. I'm very happy we've chosen a vegan diet for our family and you're here to help us keep our daughter healthy.

Certainly, don't be shy about letting the physician know if your child is "mostly vegan." Be as specific as you can. ("She eats dairy every once in a while," or "We allow her to make her own food choices whether to eat dairy or eggs when with friends," etc.) Be prepared to answer any questions the doctor may have. He may want to do a simple blood draw initially or annually to test for certain deficiencies, like B_{12}, iron, or zinc. View the physician's perhaps overly cautious approach as a health safeguard, not as a suspicion, and your relationship with your child's doctor won't be unnecessarily defensive.

With a positive relationship established, if your child ever encounters a health issue related or unrelated to nutrition, you'll be ready to address it with her physician without fear that being vegan will "come out." (See Chapter 9 for what to do if you do run into the unlikely event that your child develops a diet-related health problem.)

Parent Trap

If you've taken all these steps, but after a few visits, you still don't feel this particular doctor accepts your choice to be a vegan family, it's time to find a new doctor.

When you find the right doctor and you handle the subject of your child's vegan diet with openness and a partnering approach, not only will the physician likely be supportive of her diet, he may even ask you questions about childhood nutrition in the future!

Daycare and School Rules

The easiest way to find a veg-friendly daycare is through referrals from other vegan families. Or hire a child-care provider who is vegan or vegetarian herself. A daycare provider or center that accommodates children with food allergies will also likely respect a vegan child's special restrictions.

You may have to spell out exactly what being vegan means to the provider: no meat, no eggs, no dairy. Believe it or not, some people still think chicken isn't meat. Or that liquid egg substitute isn't really eggs. Be sure to bring in vegan snacks or a special dessert for your child's care providers every now and again to show that you value their work and you appreciate that they respect your requests.

Finding a vegan-friendly child-care provider is very similar to finding a daycare that's supportive of breast-feeding. So if you've breast-fed and established a good child-care provider at that stage, you're probably already with a respectful provider who will support your vegan choice for your new eater. If not, you've already gone through a similar process once and know you're looking for …

Trust: Do you feel you can trust this person/organization to follow your instructions? Intuition plays in here.

That's So Vegan

For an excellent step-by-step resource on how to choose a quality child-care provider, go to www.babycenter.com/0_how-to-find-good-daycare_5924.bc. Add your own questions about whether they'll adhere to your child's special dietary needs.

Open communication: Does the child-care provider send notes home daily to let parents know what the child ate, how much she slept and went to the bathroom (depending on age), and any significant happenings of the day? Or do you get time at pickup for a verbal re-cap, at least? Do you have the opportunity to write down instructions for them and ways to know they have been followed?

Open access: Can you drop in at any time to see how things are going for your child? This is critically important. If you show up unannounced, are you greeted with enthusiasm or like you're intruding? If you show up one day and your child is drinking a carton of milk and eating cheese sticks, after you've been clear she doesn't eat dairy, you can be quite certain that you need to re-assert your expectations or find another daycare.

When she's out of daycare and into school, you'll want to talk to her teacher about food in the classroom at the beginning of the school year. Because of the prevalence of childhood food allergies and religious pluralism, most schools are used to accommodating food restriction requests. Be sure to ask if there's an established policy on accommodating food restrictions if you get any resistance from the classroom teacher.

Depending on where you live and how the school is operated, your requests may be different. It's common for classrooms in some parts of the nation to pass around milk to children in lower grades at snack time. Other schools have one child bring a snack to share with the entire class. Sometimes, teachers allow parents to bring in birthday cake or cupcakes and ice cream the week of their child's birthday. It's important for the teacher to know—and to let you know ahead of time—that your child will need a snack or treat alternative.

Help your child feel comfortable about being vegan in a nonvegan school environment by asking her if she'd like to bring a treat in for her class. Read books to her about other vegan kids. The heartwarming book *Benji Beansprout Doesn't Eat Meat* author Sarah Rudy tells the story of a grade school–age boy who does just that.

That's So Vegan

The Physicians Committee for Responsible Medicine's Health School Lunch Revolution campaign hopes to encourage Congress to include veg choices in lunchrooms around the nation. CHOICE (Consumers for Healthy Options in Children's Education) is another organization that works to improve school lunches. Find out how you can support these campaigns at www.pcrm.org and www.choiceusa.net.

It's reassuring to feel that your child's daycare or school is respectful of veganism … and unsettling if you don't. Some vegan families choose to not involve their children in traditional daycare settings and instead homeschool their children. These choices may avoid conflicts in traditionally nonvegan environments, making life easier in many ways and more complicated in others. Whatever your family's choice, you can be proud that every time you speak up for your child's needs, you make it easier for the next vegan family in that situation.

The Least You Need to Know

♦ Give your picky eater the three C's: choices, control, and creativity.

♦ If you're vegan and your child's other parent is not, discuss your concerns calmly, be willing to compromise, set some boundaries, and agree to respectfully disagree.

♦ Seek the right doctor for your family until you find a good fit. Be honest up front so you can trust each other, and work together to create a positive relationship.

♦ Communicate openly, confidently, and with a listening ear when discussing your child's diet with a relative, physician, daycare provider, or school official. The more relaxed and less defensive you are, the more likely the interaction will go well.

Chapter 4

Debunking Myths About Vegan Kids

In This Chapter

- The truth behind the myths
- Health myths disproved
- Social myths set straight

Every now and again, a TV medical drama runs the malnourished vegan kid storyline. While this inexcusable situation has occurred in a few instances, it's far from the experience of most vegan families. And most of the myths about raising vegan kids you'll encounter in daily life aren't as extreme as "Your child will starve." That doesn't make them any less bothersome, however.

Common misunderstandings about veganism for kids are thrown around because of TV dramas, as well as a lack of understanding about nutrition basics, and, we believe, the general non-vegan public's assumption that vegan parents are forcing their way of life onto their young kids. (The same could be said for omnivorous parents, but we digress ....)

Most myths, however, are based on the honest belief that growing kids' extra nutritional needs simply cannot be met if they don't eat animal products. Many nonvegans think the vegan choice is fine for full-grown adults but not for growing kids. That's all bunk, and this chapter's all about getting the bunk out.

Health Myths

Vegan parents often hear the same complaints from naysayers about vegan diets for kids. In the following sections, we'll introduce those common falsehoods and give you concrete information to refute the uninformed claims.

Myth: Vegan Kids Are Weak and Sickly

Fact: Vegan kids are just as healthy, and most likely often healthier, than their omnivorous counterparts.

Parents, when confronted with this myth, stand on the 2004 report about vegan diets for kids published by *Pediatrics in Review,* the American Academy of Pediatrics journal considered top of the heap in medical information for kids' health. This journal's report called "Vegan Diets in Infants, Children and Adolescents," clearly stated: "Multiple experts have concluded independently that vegan diets can be followed safely by infants and children without compromise of nutrition or growth and with some notable health benefits." (See Chapter 1 for a complete discussion of those benefits.)

The article mentions the need for B_{12} supplementation (which you may also want to mention to cut the naysayer's next question off at the pass), which is a very simple addition to an overall very health-promoting diet.

Brendan Brazier, Canadian vegan Ironman triathlete and author of *The Thrive Diet,* talks in his book about the reactions he received from the athletic community when he began eating vegan in the 1990s: "I was told by several trainers and coaches that I would need to make a decision: I could either eat a plant-based diet *or* I could be an athlete."

Brazier, as well as vegan and vegetarian athletes such as ultra-runner Scott Jurek; all-star pro-baseball player 5'11", 270-pound Prince Fielder; tennis great Martina Navratilova; and Olympian Carl Lewis have broken the record on this myth. With strong vegan athletes like that on his side, your little athlete can feel comfortable telling any soccer coach about why he brings orange slices instead of string cheese for the team snack at half time.

Myth: You'll Stunt Your Child's Growth

Fact: There is no evidence of failure to grow in vegan children, and the slight differences in height and weight in vegan kids may actually be beneficial.

While there aren't a lot of studies currently completed on the growth of vegan kids, the *Pediatrics in Review* article cites two that show no significant growth problems. One study of 404 children in Tennessee showed "small though significant" differences in height for children younger than 5 and an average difference in weight of about 3 pounds (1.1 kilograms) less than National Center for Health Statistics norms. In another study in Britain, vegan boys were "slightly lighter and shorter" than nonvegan boys, and girls tended to weigh slightly less.

Here's the kicker: the same article says, "Smaller size may be associated with better long-term health, as has been demonstrated in animal studies." (The unfortunate irony that animal studies proved better health for vegan kids in this instance is noted but doesn't nullify the point.)

Vegan Voices

Our extended family gathered to celebrate Christmas and several of the older members of the family made comments about my daughter not eating meat, saying her growth would be stunted. I pointed at my 5'8" 12-year-old [who] has never eaten meat and jokingly said that we had quite the opposite effect ...!

—Vegan mom of two

Myth: Kids Need Meat for Protein

Fact: Plant protein sources can provide plenty of protein.

For many years, the idea that proteins from plants had to be "properly combined" was the conventional wisdom. But that has been largely discredited as unnecessary in both child and adult veg diets. In her later books, veg guru and *Diet for a Small Planet* author Francis Moore Lappé expressed regret about previously writing about properly combining plant proteins, suggesting that the concept had become too focused upon as a reason why nutritious veg diets are perceived as difficult.

Because plant proteins are about 85 percent digestible, vegan kids' diets do need a bit of a protein boost (about 2 to 14 grams more, depending upon weight and age), "which can easily be met in a diet providing adequate energy," according to the *Journal of the American Dietetic Association.*

Excellent, kid-friendly sources of protein are readily available in the plant world. Tofu, seitan, tempeh, nut butters, nuts, seeds, and beans in all shapes, sizes, and consistencies are the old standbys. Add to those today's processed soy-based meat analog creations like veggie burgers, soy sausage patties, veggie bacon, tofu hot dogs, and more (to be enjoyed in moderation), and your kids have endless animal-free protein sources.

Myth: Fish Is the Only Source for Top-Quality Omega-3s

Fact: Omega-3 fatty acids/DHA (docosahexaenoic acid) can be acquired through nonanimal sources as well as fish.

People don't need to eat fish to get omega-3s/DHA, the essential fatty acid that promises all sorts of body and brain benefits in both children and adults. Where do fish get their omega-3s? The answer is sea algae, and humans can get omega-3s the same way, and without eating a single fish.

We caution against the sole use of flaxseeds, flax oil, and a number of other nut oils for your vegan child's only source of omega-3s. They are rich in ALA (alpalinolenic acid) but deficient in DHA. The body tries to convert enough ALA to DHA, which is essential for the healthy development of your child's vision, but is not able to do so adequately enough. Some good omega-3/DHA vegan supplements from sea plant sources are available. Ask your pediatrician or family medicine doctor if your child should be supplemented.

Myth: Dairy Is the Best Source of Vitamin D and Calcium

Fact: Milk is supplemented with vitamin D, so taking a vitamin D supplement is the best source and skips the middleman—or cow, in this instance. Calcium is available from many plant products and in supplemented orange juice.

Vitamin D isn't actually a vitamin at all; it functions as a hormone used in the human body. D is a hot letter in health news lately because all the sunscreen we're wearing and kids' lack of playtime is creating a widespread case of vitamin D deficiency.

One of the best ways for your child to get vitamin D is through limited but regular sun exposure, even just 10 minutes a day on exposed, nonsunscreened, skin. A good vitamin D supplement helps eliminate any further D-deficiency worries. It's true that most vitamin D supplements are derived from animal products, but look for a vegan option or go for the BPO.

Calcium is also widely available in fortified orange juice as well as leafy greens, tofu, and some beans.

> **That's So Vegan**
>
> For more information on calcium and vitamin D, check out www.notmilk.com.

Social Myths

Now let's address the social myths, such as whether it's medically reportable child abuse to feed your child a vegan diet. Also, can vegan foods adequately replace the "joys" of the standard American diet for kids? Is an American childhood complete without ice cream, hot dogs, and mac and cheese?

Myth: Veganism Is Child Abuse

Fact: Veganism in itself is not child abuse. It has the potential to be healthy or harmful, just as does an omnivorous diet, depending on the parents' level of nutrition education, motivation, and concern for the child's welfare.

One study that focused on child neglect reports related to "complimentary therapies" lists a few unfortunate instances of meat-free diets being reported to authorities. These, however, were far from the typical vegan child's diet. One of the cases involved restrictive dietary practices where the child was allowed to eat only uncooked fruits, grains, and vegetables and, as a result, starved to death. Another involved a 20-month-old boy whose parents refused to feed him anything other than lettuce and watermelon because they thought he was a religious prophet.

Parent Trap _____

Doctors and other health-care providers are legally required to report signs of abuse and neglect. If your child is having a diet-related health problem, partner with your child's physician. No one wants to see a child off the growth charts (too light or too heavy) for a prolonged period of time or with a persistent nutrient deficiency. If your child is having weight or other nutrition issues, keep good records, attend all scheduled appointments, and build trust to be sure your doctor knows you're working to correct the problem. (See Chapter 9 for more details.)

It's not usually necessary to assume that a doctor's questions about your child's diet are an attack on veganism or your family's choices. When an omnivorous child's parents feed him foods full of saturated fat, cholesterol-laden meat, and too few fruits and vegetables, most doctors will direct as many or more questions and concerns toward those parents as they will if they sense vegan parents aren't watching out for potential pitfalls to their child's health. Whether it's too much of a bad thing, not enough of a good thing, too much weight, or too little weight, it all comes down to knowing and providing for the nutritional needs of your child at each age and stage, whether you feed him animal products or not.

Myth: Vegan Kids Are Lunchroom Bully Targets

Fact: Schools are rapidly improving both lunchroom offerings and anti-bullying policies. With the variety of portable vegan foods, your child's lunchbox can look nearly identical to his omnivorous classmates', if so desired.

Your child can fit into the lunchroom scene in so many delicious ways (see Chapter 3 for more details). And if he wants to be more open about his animal compassion through vegan eating, the lunchroom may be a good place to practice putting his beliefs out there quietly, in a natural way, by example.

Case in point: one neighborhood public school our second daughter attended was surprisingly progressive in the lunchroom. It always offered meatless options, including peanut butter and jelly and salad (her favorite). In first grade, she began to bring about half of her week's lunches from home and the other half we would pay for school lunch. We were pleasantly surprised to find out she had become known among her friends in the lunchroom as the go-to veg girl for meat identification. The kids who were animal lovers and who were interested in learning but weren't taught at home what a hamburger or pepperoni was really made from naturally gravitated to her to ask what was "okay" for them to eat in the lunch line. As they walked through the line pointing to the offerings, our daughter would give the thumbs-up for the meatless choices and shake her head "no" for animal-based foods.

In the unfortunate circumstance that your child is being bullied, however, you must intervene. Talk to your child about ideas for how to handle the problem; read books like *The Bully, the Bullied, and the Bystander: From Preschool to High School—How Parents and Teachers Can Help Break the Cycle of Violence* by Barbara Coloroso; and talk to school officials. Bullying can create life-long emotional scars and turn a child off from any difference in his life the bully may use against him, including veganism. You may not be able to prevent every act of bullying, and almost every child experiences it at some point. But don't allow it to be a prolonged pain in your child's life.

In the lunchroom, your child can make a difference both by example of what you pack from home, and with dollar power by buying school lunch and choosing the veg choices.

Myth: Vegan Kids Are Party Outcasts

Fact: Many kids with food restrictions due to allergies, diabetes, religion, and other issues are actively involved in all sorts of youth activities. Nothing about veganism inherently prevents your child from participating in any activity.

Parties and other group events like scouting, sports, church activities, and after-school programs bring fun and camaraderie—and often nonvegan food—into your child's life. There's no need to avoid any of them because he's vegan. Accommodate the food needs, and focus on the fun.

Let's look at birthday parties, for example. The easiest birthday party to attend for vegan kids is, of course, their own. Not only can the cake and food be vegan, but it's a great opportunity to introduce the invitees to the great taste of animal-product-free foods and the joys of animal compassion. At her eleventh birthday party, our oldest daughter opted to share her love of animals in need with her invited friends by asking them to bring food and toy donations for the local animal shelter in lieu of gifts for her.

Going to other kids' nonvegan parties needn't be a problem, either, especially if you and your child know the birthday child's family well and they know you're vegan. In all honesty, a few acquaintances or classmates might not invite your child to a birthday party because he's vegan (or invite your family to a cookout for the same reason). This is a sad reality of a subset of close-minded stragglers who simply haven't caught up with the times to know that vegans aren't outcasts and can actually assimilate just fine at a party full of omnivores. We hope and assume they are the exception, not the rule, in most communities today.

> **Vegan Voices**
>
> Always bring the best available vegan organic cake to their friends' birthday parties, so that all the kids will want a slice of your children's vegan cake.
>
> —Aviram, India

Explain to the parent hosting the party that your child is vegan and you need to bring a bit of something for him to eat. It's fine to bring a little vegan cake (like Amy's Kitchen Organic Chocolate or Orange cakes) or cupcakes to provide something for your child to eat at cake time, and maybe a little something to share. (But be sure it's not as pretty or as big as the birthday child's cake! You don't want to detract from the reason for the party.)

As for other events, it seems like a lot of scouting, church groups, and sports teams events are focused on nonvegan food—cookie sales, pancake and sausage breakfasts, candy sales, pizza sales, pizza parties, cookouts, and camping weekends that contain lots of meaty meals. With your help, your vegan child can participate in almost all these events (minus the sales, perhaps—consider making a donation instead). Help social events be more vegan-friendly for your child by ...

- Bringing your own veg food, including enough to pass around to others when appropriate.

- Joining organizations that are more veg-friendly. Jane Goodall's worldwide group for kids with local chapters called Roots and Shoots (www.rootsandshoots.org) is an alternative option to scouting.

- Hosting events for sports teams, youth groups, or church events at your home. Sure, it takes more work, but when it's at your home, you can set the menu, know where your child is, and get to know his friends better.

- Focusing on other aspects of the event and leaving the food portion out. If it's a cookout, go out to eat at your favorite veg-friendly restaurant beforehand and show up for the games, for example.

Myth: You're Depriving Them of Childhood Fun

Fact: Health is fun. Being compassionate toward animals is fun. Saving the environment is fun.

One dad in our vegan parents' survey put it this way:

My child doesn't see veganism as limiting or restrictive. He sees it as interesting and a challenge. We make vegan food an exciting thing in our house. His school and society have taught him how fragile and beautiful our environment is ... when he remembers his childhood, he will remember it with fondness and a special passion to make this world a little bit better.

That doesn't sound like deprivation, does it?

Yet some people your child interacts with (including parents like ourselves in the anxious "Am I a good parent?" moments that we all face, vegan or not) will have some lingering questions about the traditional baseball game hot dog, the birthday cake, the ice-cream cones, and the Thanksgiving turkey (with wishbone). How can a child grow up without experiencing these food-based cultural memories?

He doesn't have to. There's a vegan substitute for all those sentimental favorites and more—right down to a wishbone in the tofu-turkey. What's more, some professional baseball stadiums like Yankee Stadium have begun to sell tofu dogs.

Myth: Vegan Food Can't Taste Good

Fact: From the most elegant restaurant to the best backyard barbecue, vegan food rivals any culinary tradition.

This myth may very well have been true if we were writing this book in 1981. But thanks to dedicated entrepreneurs, talented chefs, creative cookbook authors, and the natural foods movement, veganism has come a long way.

Consider tofu, for example. Once known as a white, tasteless blob that was only edible drowned in soy sauce, tofu now comes baked, fried, cubed, marinated, and more.

Restaurants like the Candle Cafe in New York City showcase gourmet vegan cuisine. Vegan bakeries churn out cupcakes, wedding cakes, and amazing pastries that are either hard to distinguish from or better than their egg-, butter-, and cream cheese–laden cousins. Vegan chocolates? Of course. And as you'll see in Part 4, today's vegan family can eat delicious, affordable vegan meals any night of the week.

The Least You Need to Know

- Infants and children can follow vegan diets safely without compromising nutrition or growth—and with some notable health benefits.

- Current studies suggest that vegan kids may be slightly smaller than their omnivorous counterparts. Smaller size may be associated with better long-term health.

- Take advantage of the excellent, kid-friendly sources of protein, vitamins, and minerals in the plant world. Whatever nutrient needs a boost in your child's diet can be achieved by taking a supplement. Vegan kids' diets do need a bit of a protein boost.

- The lunchroom, birthday parties, and baseball games don't have to be avoided. Vegan kids can fit in, have fun, and maintain their food ethics in any of these social situations.

- Social myths that vegan families are neglectful, depriving, tasteless, or isolated can be easily countered with education; creativity; and a fun, open attitude.

Part 2

Nutritional Needs of Vegan Kids

A plant-based vegan diet is an incredibly healthful choice for kids, as long as special nutritional needs—such as vitamin B_{12} and a handful of other vitamins, minerals, and nutrients—are met. Parents can readily meet these special needs with some basic nutrition information, an awareness of kids' unique growth and development needs at different ages, and a commitment to meeting their child's needs even when the child throws them a curve ball—hello, picky eater.

The vast majority of vegan kids eat an extraordinarily healthful diet compared to their counterparts eating the standard American diet. Part 2 helps ensure that you're optimizing your child's diet to provide everything she needs to thrive.

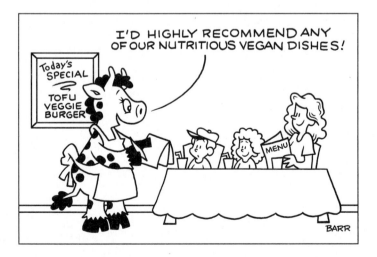

5

Vegan Babies (0 to 12 Months)

In This Chapter

- ◆ Help your doctor help your baby
- ◆ Human milk for human babies
- ◆ When it's time for solids
- ◆ A baby-appropriate meal plan

Every day, babies bring smiles, love, and *worry* into a parent's life. Everything has to be just perfect for your little wonder, including what she eats.

In this chapter, we talk about how to be sure your baby gets the healthiest nutritional start possible. Find out how to partner with her doctor and be her spokesperson in medical situations. All the vegan-specific info you need about baby nutritional needs, favorite food lists, and safe eating tips are here, too. We also include a sample meal plan specifically for the newest vegans.

Tune in to your baby's individual personality, learn about her vegan-specific nutritional needs, and get comfortable with change (which will happen almost daily in these stages of childhood growth). This is the start of a very long and beautiful growing season for your little sprout.

Be Your Baby's Medical Spokesperson

Especially when your child is too young to speak for herself, it's up to you to help your doctor help her. Make it to all the regularly scheduled well-baby visits. This not only ensures your child is hitting all the appropriate milestones, but also helps you create a relationship with your child's doctor when all is well. When your child is sick, the more information you can bring to her doctor, the easier it will be for the doctor to make a correct diagnosis and the quicker your little one can be 100 percent healthy again.

It's also important to keep good records of your child's health history and medical information. Doctors are extremely busy, and your child will likely see many different health-care professionals in most clinics. Be your child's medical advocate to ensure the best, most error-free health care possible. At each appointment, bring the bottles of any medications she's currently taking, including vitamins and other supplements (herbal, etc.), whether over-the-counter or prescription. Bring a copy of your child's immunization records, too, so there's no confusion about whether she needs to receive one at this visit. Write a list of questions you have beforehand so you don't forget to ask anything. At most clinics, doctors typically have about 15 minutes per appointment, so they need you to focus on the most important issues for this visit.

Parent Trap

A note on vaccines: because many vaccines are not vegan (and for many other reasons), some parents are choosing not to have their kids fully vaccinated, which is against current standard medical practice. For a more in-depth discussion of this topic and an alternative vaccine schedule, see *The Vaccine Book* by Dr. Robert Sears, and talk to your doctor about any concerns you have.

If you have any concerns related to your child's diet or food-related health problems (constipation, diarrhea, allergies, hyperactivity, headaches, weight loss, being overweight, or slow growth, for example) be sure to keep a log of what and approximately how much she eats for a few days prior to the appointment to help your doctor clue in on possible causes.

If your child sees complementary health professionals such as a homeopath, naturopath, dietician, acupuncturist, or chiropractor, it's important to let them know she's vegan, too. Anecdotally, most of the professionals who work in complementary or alternative therapies are more open to vegan diets. However, as integrative medicine takes hold in mainstream Western medicine, more M.D.s and D.O.s seem to be accepting of (if not personally enthusiastic about) veganism.

Breast Is Best

Human milk is the only kind of mammalian milk on which little people were made to thrive and grow. If you've ever wondered why eating too many full-fat dairy products can make people overweight, look at how quickly babies grow on human breast milk! Breast milk makes babies grow nice and chubby quickly to give them reserves in case of illness and on which to grow strong and lean as they go through the energetic toddler years.

The American Academy of Pediatrics (AAP) and the American Academy of Family Physicians (AAFP) both recommend breast-feeding as the best form of infant nutrition. Breast-feeding your baby is the easiest way to ensure she is getting the best start in life. Breast milk has all the nutrients a baby needs, antibodies to guard against infection, and healthy fats to promote brain development. In addition to the nutritional benefits, breast-feeding requires proper

That's So Vegan

Vegan moms' breast milk is lower in environmental pollutants, including DDT (dichlorodiphenyltrichloroethane), chlordane, and PCBs (polychlorinated biphenyls), according to a study published in the *New England Journal of Medicine*. In most cases, levels were just 1 or 2 percent of those seen in the general population.

jaw motion for mouth and teeth formation, and it promotes healthy emotional attachment between mother and baby. And there's a whole host of long-term protective health benefits, including reduced risk for female cancers and diabetes, for breast-feeding mothers as well.

Many new moms say that the early days and weeks (sometimes even months) of breast-feeding are like riding a roller coaster: fun one moment, screams the next. You need support to get through problems that may arise. The best place to start is the La Leche League (www. lalecheleague.org or 1-877-4-LA-LECHE [1-877-452-5324]). There you'll find free, mother-to-mother breast-feeding information and support. Almost any breast-feeding problem can be overcome. The lifelong health rewards for you and for your baby are worth the effort.

The AAP recommends all babies be exclusively breast-fed for the first 6 months of life and then to continue for at least another 12 months while introducing solids, or as long as is mutually agreeable between mom and baby.

What's more, breast-feeding moms who eat a varied, healthful, and multiflavored diet—all hallmarks of a good vegan diet—often find their children have more adventurous tastes and gravitate toward healthier foods.

Nutrition for Breast-Feeding Vegans

Vegan moms take note: if you're breast-feeding, in many ways, you're still eating for two. In particular, be extra vigilant about taking your *vitamin B_{12}* supplement daily because breast-fed babies of vegan moms can become deficient in this vitamin. In fact, the babies can be deficient *without the mom ever showing signs of a deficiency herself.* Vitamin B_{12} is a crucial nutrient for a baby's healthy brain growth and function. In the case of most nutrients, even in famine conditions, the mother's body will rob her own supplies to provide the baby with needed nutrients. But not in the case of B_{12}.

> **Vegan Vocab**
>
> Vitamin B_{12} is an important nutrient for red blood cell formation and for healthy nerve tissues. Deficiencies can lead to anemia and permanent nerve and brain damage.

Yet it's simple to prevent this and other deficiencies. After the baby is born, continue to take your prenatal multivitamin daily. More is not better in the case of vitamins, so don't overdo it. Take vitamins that supply the 100 percent recommended daily allowance or less. Fat-soluble vitamins like A and E are secreted in human milk and could cause liver toxicity in the baby if mom takes too high a dose.

Also, eat about 500 calories more a day than you would if you weren't pregnant or nursing. (That's equivalent to a peanut butter and jelly sandwich on 2 slices of whole-wheat bread, 20 dried apricots, or a couple handfuls of mixed nuts.) Be sure you don't drop below 1,800 calories a day no matter what.

Is Your Breast-Fed Baby Getting Enough?

In our culture that likes to quantify everything, it can be initially unsettling that breasts don't come with little liquid measuring marks indicating how many ounces are in there for your baby at any given time.

But like most things in nature, it's not quite as straightforward as measuring ounces. In fact, lactating breasts are almost constantly in the state of milk production, and most moms will feel milk "let down" more than once during a feeding.

Additionally, if the nursing mother is working and pumping breast milk for other caregivers to feed the baby in a bottle during work hours, or if she is supplementing breast milk with formula, the amount of breast milk will adjust. And if you continue to breast-feed past the 6-month mark after solid foods are introduced, breast milk becomes one of many food choices, so the amount and frequency of nursing sessions changes dramatically and varies greatly from one mother-baby pair to another. It comes down to simple economics: demand equals supply.

Once you get the hang of it, knowing if your baby is getting enough breast milk usually comes naturally. Especially in the early months, there are some general rules of thumb to follow. According to the La Leche League:

◆ In the early weeks and months, your baby should nurse about 8 to 12 times a day.

◆ Typically during the first few days, she will wet only one or two diapers a day.

◆ After mother's milk comes in, usually on the third or fourth day, the baby should begin to have 6 to 8 wet cloth diapers (5 or 6 wet disposable diapers) per day. (An easy way to feel the weight of a wet disposable diaper is to pour 2 to 4 tablespoons water in a dry diaper.)

◆ Most young babies will have at least 2 to 5 bowel movements every 24 hours for the first several months, although some babies will switch to less frequent but larger bowel movements at about 6 weeks.

◆ Watch the baby, not the clock. Let the baby nurse as often as she wants as long as she will.

◆ Babies may lose a few ounces in the first few days after birth. This is normal. But babies should gain at least 4 to 7 ounces per week after the fourth day of life.

© *La Leche League International, October 2008.*

If you have any concerns about weight gain or feeding patterns, contact your physician or a local lactation consultant. (Most pediatricians and family medicine physicians allow you to bring your baby in for a weight check free of charge.)

In the first 6 months, if your baby is generally content, alert, and active; appears healthy; has good color and firm skin; has the recommended output of urine and bowel movements; and is growing, you can be sure she is getting all the nutrition she needs from you.

The Formula Option

If a vegan baby is not breast-feeding, the only option in infant formula is soy formula. This falls under the BPO (best possible option) category. Currently, artificial infant formulas of any kind aren't as healthy as breast milk in many ways. No soy formulas are approved for preterm infant use, so if your baby is a preemie, it's breast-feeding or milk-based formula. And almost all soy formulas reportedly contain some animal-based products from the vitamin D supplement in the formula (derived from sheep wool or bird feather extract).

This all points back to encouraging vegan moms to work through any hesitations about or complications during breast-feeding. But for the limited number of moms who truly cannot breast-feed, soy infant formula or milk-based formula in the case of premature babies is the current BPO.

That said, soy formula may increase the risk of babies developing peanut allergies. There's no evidence to confirm that the phytoestrogen and isoflavones in soy may affect the growth or hormonal balance of developing human babies, but it's an ongoing field of study because those components have been shown to have effects on animals.

On the plus side, soy formula has been shown to reduce the duration of diarrhea in babies experiencing gastroenteritis. But even then, after that illness is gone, the AAP recommends parents return to breast milk or cow's-milk-based formula.

If you feed your baby soy formula, be sure to follow the recommended feeding schedules and preparation recipe for the individual brand you have. Be aware that formula-fed babies will have fewer bowel movements because formula tends to be constipating, but still watch urine and bowel movement output and visit your child's doctor for regular well-baby checkups and weight gain checks.

Your pediatrician or family medicine physician may question your choice of soy formula. Be honest about your reasons and open about your vegan choice. AAP and AAFP guidelines tell doctors to direct parents toward breast-feeding and cow's-milk-based formulas "in most cases" but do note exceptions for babies with allergies to cow protein and "strict vegans."

When choosing how to feed your baby, keep in mind that breast-feeding or formula feeding doesn't have to be a one-or-the-other proposition. If there's a need to supplement with formula because of reduced milk supply, a work situation, or other reasons, you can still continue to breast-feed. Identify your goals for feeding your baby, get support as necessary, and adjust as needed. Many moms who set a goal to breast-feed their baby for 3 months find themselves still nursing the baby at a year. Some moms who plan to wean at a year end up allowing their toddler to naturally wean themselves over a period of many months.

Parent Trap _____

Never use regular soy milk to feed a baby. Never attempt to make homemade infant formula or buy it from a source other than major manufacturers regulated by the FDA. As the infant formula tragedies in China sadly proved, not including all nutrients, reducing certain levels of essential nutrients, or allowing contaminants into infant formula can cause the illness or death of otherwise perfectly healthy babies. Don't take the risk.

Introducing Solid Foods

It can be a shock the first time your sweet little baby is sitting on your lap at dinner and sticks his hand in the middle of your plate. What's he doing? Trying to give you a clue, albeit a messy one, that he's ready for solids.

Around the middle of an infant's first year, he will likely begin to show signs of readiness for solid foods—sitting up on his own, grabbing food from your plate, seeming to be hungry despite nursing as much or more than usual, and decreasing tongue thrust when food is placed in his mouth.

Now is the time to set the tone for your baby's life-long tastes in food. If babies are first introduced to solids with ice cream, cheese, and refined flour products as first foods, they'll develop a taste for creamy, high-fat foods with low-nutrient values. If babies are introduced to soy yogurt, avocados, and whole-grain foods, their palates will gravitate to naturally creamy, hearty, nutrient-dense food choices.

Most parents start their babies' solid food adventures with infant rice cereal. Often iron fortified, nonallergenic, and easy to mix with breast milk or formula, it's a good first food choice. But other premade infant foods, such as jarred baby foods, can usually be considered a waste of money. According to many baby nutrition experts, expensive premade baby foods are highly processed and some contain undesirable fillers or preservatives.

Some organic, jarred vegan baby foods are now available, and buying it in a pinch or for travel, for example, may be worth the expense, but many parents choose to make their own baby foods at home. (See *The Complete Idiot's Guide to Feeding Your Baby and Toddler* for an excellent primer on that—just bypass the meat and poultry sections.)

And during the first few weeks or months of food introduction, after allergies are ruled out, some parents become so adept at knowing what their baby likes, they feed their older baby mashed food right from their own plate to baby's mouth. This is ideal in many regards, as baby's tastes and nutrition naturally mirrors her parents' right from the start.

> **That's So Vegan**
>
> The ultra-smooth, almost artificial texture of bottled baby foods can make the transition to regular foods more difficult for some babies and doesn't help them practice grasping small foods with their own little fingers.

Beware: Choking Hazards

While you're introducing solid foods, keep this in mind: some of the healthiest foods may, unfortunately, also be choking hazards. Avoid these vegan snack choices for babies and toddlers:

- Apples with peels (serve peeled, diced small)
- Chunks of any food, like vegan cheese and tofu cubes
- Globs of peanut butter or other nut butters
- Gum
- Hard, gooey, or sticky candies
- Nuts and seeds
- Popcorn and chips
- Raisins and other dried fruit
- Raw veggies (unless grated)
- Tofu dogs (scrambled tofu or mashed tofu is okay)
- Whole grapes

Almost any fruit or veggie that can be puréed or mashed is a good choice for baby's first food. A number of manufacturers are producing great baby food, and simply using your fork or the back of your spoon to soften up and smooth out a bit of food you're eating works, too. What's on Mom's plate usually looks best to baby, so be prepared to cook for two for a while even though you're not eating for two.

Basic Nutrition for Vegan Infants

Optimal infant nutrition comes down to breast-feeding. This was once a controversial statement, but choosing not to breast-feed is no longer a preference as much as it is a risk.

According to the *Journal of the American Dietetic Association*, many vegan women continue to breast-feed their babies well past the 6-month minimum recommendation, and this is an excellent way to ensure nutrition throughout the entire first year, prior to solid food introduction and beyond. To ensure proper nutrition, babies being fed with infant formula should slowly wean off infant formula from 6 months through the first year.

The following sections offer some specific nutritional needs for your vegan infant.

Calories

Caloric intake for infants varies greatly as babies grow exponentially in the first days, weeks, and months. Even within individual feedings, breast milk caloric content changes drastically from the skim milk–like fore milk at first to the good-fat-laden hind milk at the end of a feeding.

At about 1 year, most babies need about 900 calories a day. As solid foods are introduced, choose natural foods rich in nutrients and calories.

Protein

Around 7 or 8 months, most babies have tried enough solid foods that they're ready for some of the more complex, protein-rich foods like well-mashed beans, mashed tofu, and soy yogurt.

Babies at 9 months need about 15 grams protein daily.

Vitamins and Minerals

Breast milk and fortified infant formula provide almost all the vitamins and minerals infants need. But there are a few exceptions:

Iron: If your baby eats iron-fortified infant cereals when you introduce solids and you continue to introduce other iron-rich foods as he gets older, no other iron supplementation should be necessary.

Vitamin B$_{12}$: According to the American Dietetic Association, unless vegan moms who breast-feed regularly supplement their diet with B$_{12}$, "it is important that all breast-fed vegan infants receive a regular supplement of vitamin B$_{12}$" (0.4 ug, or microgram, per day for the first 6 months, 0.5 ug/day beginning at age 6 months). B$_{12}$ deficiencies can cause irreversible brain damage and must be safeguarded against.

Vitamin D: Families who live in higher latitudes or seasonal climates or who do not get adequate sunlight outdoors regularly should provide a daily 400 IU (international units) vitamin D supplement for their vegan baby starting at about 3 months.

Vitamin K: This shot is given to most babies shortly after birth and is important to prevent uncontrolled bleeding.

Zinc: The evidence is still mixed on whether vegan babies should receive a zinc supplement. The AAP currently doesn't recommend zinc supplements for vegan infants. Guidelines from the Institute of Medicine suggest an upper limit of zinc of 5 milligrams/day for 6-month- to 1-year-old infants but a well-respected pediatric text suggests 2 milligrams for babies up to 6 months and 3 milligrams for 7 months to 4 years.

Fats/Omega-3s

DHA (docosahexaenoic acid) and EPA (eicosapentanoic acid), which are the beneficial omega-3 fats, promote healthy brain and eyesight development. No set-in-stone recommendations currently exist for how much DHA supplementation is appropriate for babies. However, leading pediatrician Dr. William Sears recommends approximately 500 milligrams a day for infants aged 6 months and older. (Dr. Sears's markets omega-3 products that are fish oil based.)

There is DHA in breast milk (although lower in vegan moms than vegetarian and omnivorous moms), and some infant formulas are supplemented with it (although the levels in the infant formulas are lower than in vegan breast-feeding moms).

Hydration

Babies up to 6 months old obviously get all their hydration needs from the food they drink—breast milk or infant formula. It's not a good idea to give babies sugar water or any other old wives' tale concoctions. (Babies' kidneys can't regulate water or water and sugar. They need to have breast milk or formula that has the proper balance of electrolytes or they can become very ill.)

After 6 months, you can add some juice and smoothies. But the AAP suggests no more than $^3/_4$ cup (4 to 6 ounces) juice a day for kids over 6 months. Look for 100 percent pasteurized juice. Another good choice is calcium-fortified orange juice because calcium is a mineral to watch in vegan diets.

> **Parent Trap**
>
> Babies under 1 year old should not be given regular soy milk. It should be supplemented with breast milk or soy infant formula until age 2 at which age the child is able to drink up to 24 ounces soy milk daily.

Sample Meal Plan for Vegan Babies

A sample meal plan for vegan infants may be the most difficult to offer because it will vary widely from family to family. Those first foods will depend on if a baby is breast-fed or formula fed, how careful a parent must be about introducing new foods because of a history of family food allergies, parents' choice to use jarred baby food, and whether the infant is in a child-care setting.

The Vegetarian Resource Group (VRG) develops and posts excellent resources for vegan infants, children, and adults at its website, vrg. org. The sample menu on the next page is from the VRG and applies to babies ages 4 to 12 months. (Overlap of ages occurs because of varying rate of development.)

Sample Menu for Babies (0 to 12 Months)

Food	4 to 6 Months	6 to 8 Months	9 to 10 Months	11 to 12 Months
Milk	Human milk or soy formula	Human milk or soy formula	Human milk or soy formula	Human milk or soy formula
Cereal and bread	Iron-fortified infant cereal (can be delayed until 6 months)	Infant cereal, crackers, toast, unsweetened dry cereal	Infant cereal, crackers, toast, unsweetened dry cereal, soft bread	Infant cereal, crackers, toast, unsweetened dry cereal, soft bread, rice, pasta
Fruits	None	Strained fruit, fruit juice	Soft or cooked fruit, fruit juice	Soft, canned or cooked fruit, peeled raw fruit, fruit juice
Vegetables	None	Strained vegetables, vegetable juice	Soft, cooked mashed vegetables, vegetable juice	Soft, cooked pieces of vegetable, vegetable juice
Legumes	None	Tofu, puréed legumes, soy yogurt (at 7 or 8 months)	Tofu, puréed legumes, soy cheese, soy yogurt	Tofu, mashed legumes, soy cheese, soy yogurt, bite-size pieces of soy burger, tempeh

Reed Mangels, Ph.D., R.D., from "Simply Vegan," by The Vegetarian Resource Group; www.vrg.org.

The Least You Need to Know

- Breast milk is the superior infant food. Most mom and baby pairs can breast-feed with the right information and support.

- If a vegan baby is not breast-feeding, the only option in infant formula is soy formula. Parents should never use soy milk as infant formula.

- Introduce solid foods around the middle of the first year. Watch for signs of readiness like grabbing for food, hungriness after nursing, and loss of tongue thrust.

- Some of the healthiest foods can be choking hazards for babies and toddlers. Watch the size, shape, and consistency of the food you serve to your infant and toddler.

Chapter 6

Vegan Toddlers (1 to 3 Years)

In This Chapter

- ◆ Breast milk: it's not just for babies
- ◆ Toddler feeding tips: what to avoid
- ◆ What busy toddlers need to thrive
- ◆ A toddler-appropriate meal plan

If a blur of light and sound twirls through your living room, darts under your bed, and squeals at your dinner table, it's likely a toddler inhabits your home. These fast-moving, babbling, risk-taking creatures are tons of fun—and work—to have around the house.

Trying to catch and feed a toddler is a challenge unto itself. When you do catch the wriggling mass, it's important to feed him the good, nutritious stuff because the toddler tongue is a palate in training. Feed him junk food, he'll develop a taste for sweet, salty, fatty foods. Feed him natural, whole foods, and he'll find artificial, refined foods far too sweet and fake tasting.

In this chapter, you catch up with your vegan toddler's nutritional needs, identify his eating danger zones, and find out why breast-feeding into toddlerhood is the best health insurance you *can't* buy, especially for vegan toddlers. We also include a sample meal plan created by an expert with The Vegetarian Resource Group. So lace up your running shoes—you're in training to catch a toddler for dinner!

Breast Milk: Vegan Toddler Health Insurance

Fewer than 40 percent of American moms breast-feed their babies past the first few months of life. Only about 5 percent of moms breast-feed their toddlers to at least 18 months. This is unfortunate because the nutrition benefits and illness prevention breast milk provides go on far into toddlerhood.

The U.S. Centers for Disease Control and Prevention set a modest goal of just 25 percent of American babies to be breast-fed to at least 1 year by 2010. Why does the federal government care that more babies breast-feed to a year or more? Because breast-fed babies save millions of health-care dollars, mean fewer lost days of work for their parents, and continue to save untold millions of dollars and thousands of lives from long-term illnesses far into adulthood. And that's for both breast-fed children and their moms because breast-feeding also reduces illnesses such as female cancers in women.

> ### That's So Vegan
>
> Vegan moms of breast-feeding vegan toddlers should continue to take a multivitamin that includes vitamin B_{12} and/or provide B_{12} supplementation for their toddler.

It's clear: breast-feeding offers protection from both short-term illnesses like colds, ear infections, and allergies, and long-term chronic health problems like obesity, diabetes, and childhood cancers.

Perhaps as important as illness protection, breast-feeding provides a way to ensure that a busy toddler takes a break from his constant exploring to nurse, which boosts daily calorie intake. Breast milk contains about 20 calories per ounce of protein, healthy fats, and other nutrients; compare that to 15 calories in 1 ounce apple juice, which is simply sugar and contains no protein or healthy fats.

Sometimes, toddlers seem to go on eating strikes, where they consume next to nothing for days. Parents of breast-feeding toddlers worry much less through these phases because rarely will a breast-feeding toddler refuse to nurse, even when sick with a cold or stomach bug. Breast-feeding is a source of physical and emotional nourishment that allows them time to quiet down, refuel, and be close to mom so they can return to exploring, rested, tanked up nutritionally, and reassured emotionally.

Toddler Eating Danger Zones

Toddlerhood is a time when new dangers come into play in many areas of daily life. Choking hazards; prolonged bottle-feeding; and reliance on nutrition-poor, flavor-heavy foods are the three food dangers to avoid most cautiously.

Choking Hazards

In Chapter 5, we presented a list of the most common food choking hazards for babies and toddlers. But it's not just *what* toddlers eat. *Where and how they eat* can contribute to choking incidents, too. Be sure your toddler doesn't eat while running, playing roughly, laying down, or strapped into his car seat in the backseat alone.

When learning to feed themselves, some toddlers get overzealous about the amount of food they put into their little mouths, especially if they really love that particular food. Remind your child often to take little bites and chew, chew, chew before swallowing to teach safer eating habits.

Continuing to Use Bottles

It's easy for parents of bottle-fed babies to continue to have their child use a bottle into toddlerhood as a get-to-sleep tool. Wean your toddler from the bottle as soon as possible because prolonged bottle use contributes to tooth decay as well as an unhealthy attachment to the bottle as an oral pacifier. If your toddler uses a bottle, give it to him only during certain times of day for supplemental formula—not for juices—and not at nap- or bedtime.

Nutrition-Poor, Flavor-Heavy Foods

Now is the time to shape your child's palate toward healthy vegan eating by presenting foods that are as whole, natural, and healthful as possible. He'll be introduced to junk food soon enough by extended family, friends, and school, so it's important to set the tone now while you're still in control of your child's daily eating.

Heavily salted, overly sugared, or deep-fried foods, as well as artificial colors and flavors, are the main no-no's to avoid.

Here are some simple ways to avoid salt:

◆ Use low-sodium vegetable stock and low-sodium soy sauce

◆ Rinse canned beans

◆ Buy natural, no-salt-added peanut butter and unsalted nuts

◆ Choose low-sodium canned soups

◆ Eliminate potato chips and other salty snack foods from your toddler's choices

Parent Trap

If your child is sensitive to artificial colors and flavors, his mood will show it. In *The NDD™ Book,* pediatrician William Sears recommends keeping a "food-mood" journal so you can track what foods affect your child's behavior.

When you do use salt, choose iodized because iodine is essential to your child's health.

Reducing the amount of sugary foods your toddler consumes starts with limiting juices and chocolate soy milk, dried fruits, and sugary desserts. Of course, toddlers should completely forego sodas and candy of all kinds.

Basic Nutrition for Vegan Toddlers

Talk with your toddler's doctor about his vegan diet. Consider keeping a food journal for a week to help you reflect on his eating patterns rather than obsessively worrying about perfect nutritional balance at every meal, which will rarely happen in toddlerhood.

If he's a picky eater or going through one of the particularly sparse eating phases so common to toddlers, his doctor may recommend a daily multivitamin or particular supplement to meet his needs in this time of rapid growth and development.

Calories

Most experts agree that toddlers should eat about 1,000 to 1,500 calories per day, give or take a little depending on his size and activity level. For vegan toddlers, getting too many calories should not be an issue as long as fruit juices, a major source of calories, are limited to perhaps once or twice a day.

Of more concern is making sure the toddler meets his minimum calorie needs, especially when he goes through a phase of disinterest in food. As mentioned earlier, continuing to breast-feed helps during these times. Especially if he's not nursing, be sure he eats as many nutritionally sound and calorie-rich foods as possible, try to find enriched foods he likes, and talk to your doctor about an appropriate multivitamin. On days when he wants to eat very little, focus on calorie-dense foods like avocadoes, bananas, fortified soy and nut milks, whole grains, and (for older toddlers) thinly spread nut butters.

Protein

According to the American Dietetic Association, vegan toddlers ages 1 through 3 should consume 18 to 21 grams protein per day. This is higher than the recommended amount of daily protein for nonvegan children by about 5 to 7 grams because of the digestibility of plant-based proteins.

A serving of 2 tablespoons hummus, 1 cup soy milk, or $^2/_3$ cup pasta provides those extra 5 to 7 grams.

Vitamins

At all ages, vitamin B_{12} is the most important vitamin for vegan parents to be aware of in their child's nutritional profile. Cereals, soy milk, and nutritional yeasts supplemented with B_{12} are all good options. A daily children's multivitamin supplement is an easy way to take care of the B_{12} issue for your toddler. (See the "Important Recommended Daily Nutrients" table in Chapter 9 for nutrition requirement specifics and supplement recommendations.)

Other vitamins, including vitamin D, riboflavin, vitamin C, vitamin A, and the other B-complex vitamins can be easily acquired through a whole foods, diverse vegan diet that includes fortified toddler-friendly foods like cereals and soy milk, and a generally healthful family lifestyle, such as moderate sun exposure for proper vitamin D synthesis.

Minerals

Calcium, iron, and zinc are the "Big Three" minerals to watch in vegan children's diets.

Calcium: Children ages 1 to 3 years should get about 500 milligrams calcium each day. Just 1 cup of most calcium-fortified soy milks provides about 400 milligrams calcium. Tofu, leafy greens, and calcium-fortified orange juices are also good sources of calcium for vegan toddlers.

Parent Trap

Vitamins containing iron are one of the leading causes of childhood poisoning. If you have iron-containing vitamins in your home, take every caution to keep the safety lid tightly on the bottle and store it safely out of reach of your toddler. Tell your toddler in a way he can understand that he must only eat a vitamin when mommy or daddy gives it to him and that it could make him very, very sick if he ate more than one a day.

Iron: Parents of vegan toddlers should be extra careful about iron intake, because iron stores from babyhood are depleting; toddlers are likely not eating iron-fortified baby cereal any longer; and a lot of iron-rich vegan foods, like spinach, aren't toddler favorites. When your child does eat iron-rich foods, such as beans, raisins, or iron-fortified breakfast cereals, consider serving them with a glass of orange juice, as vitamin C helps with iron absorption.

Zinc: Because the most common sources of zinc in diets are from meat and eggs, zinc is a concern for vegan children. Protein helps zinc become more *bioavailable* in the body, so try to feed your toddler foods rich in both. Still, the human body has more trouble using zinc from plant foods when it also ingests large amounts of whole grains and legumes, often high in vegan diets.

Vegan Vocab

A vitamin's or mineral's **bioavailablity** means the amount of the substance the human body can actually use. This can vary depending on many factors including what other vitamins, minerals, and nutrients are eaten with it.

The American Dietetic Association recommends that parents of vegan children who eat a lot of cereals and legumes consider a supplement containing zinc, "especially in early childhood."

Sample Meal Plan for Vegan Toddlers

Stay flexible with your toddler's diet. As long as you set the baseline with healthful food choices, feed him whenever he says he's hungry, and/or offer food many times a day, your vegan toddler will likely develop good eating habits that will serve him well throughout life.

Sample Meal Plan for Vegan Toddlers (1 to 3 Years)

Food Group	Number of Servings
Grains	6 or more servings (A serving is ½ to 1 slice bread; ¼ to ½ cup cooked cereal, grain, or pasta; ½ to ¾ cup ready-to-eat cereal.)
Legumes, nuts, seeds	2 or more servings (A serving is ¼ to ½ cup cooked beans, tofu, tempeh, or TVP; 1½ to 3 ounces meat analog; 1 or 2 tablespoons nuts, seeds, or nut or seed butter.)
Fortified soy milk, etc.	3 servings (A serving is 1 cup fortified soy milk, infant formula, or breast milk.)
Vegetables	2 or more servings (A serving is ¼ to ½ cup cooked or ½ to 1 cup raw vegetables.)
Fruits	3 or more servings (A serving is ¼ to ½ cup canned fruit; ½ cup juice; or 1 medium fruit.)
Fats	3 servings (A serving is 1 teaspoon margarine or oil; use ½ teaspoon flaxseed oil or 2 teaspoons canola oil daily to supply omega-3 fatty acids.)

Reed Mangels, Ph.D., R.D., from "Simply Vegan," by The Vegetarian Resource Group; www.vrg.org.

The Least You Need to Know

◆ Vegan moms should be encouraged to breast-feed their vegan toddlers and continue to take a B_{12} supplement themselves.

◆ Parents of toddlers need to watch for choking hazards and poor food choices that train their children's palates to like extra-sweet, salty, fatty foods.

◆ Wean a bottle-fed toddler to a cup as early as possible. Limit the amount of juice given via bottle or cup.

◆ Feeding your toddler nutritious, healthful foods now helps your child develop a taste for the good stuff.

Vegan Kids (4 to 8 Years)

In This Chapter

◆ Pick your food battles wisely

◆ Tips for dealing with eating challenges

◆ Meeting vegan kids' nutrition needs

◆ A kid-appropriate meal plan

Once kids leave behind toddlerhood, they begin to interface with the larger, nonvegan world on their own to a much greater degree. When your child is in school, at friends' homes, or in after-school activities and sports, the ability to make her own food choices depends largely on how she feels about being vegan, how much she knows about where different foods come from, and how much she has learned (or retained) about basic nutrition.

If your family has eaten a vegan diet for as long as your child can remember, making pro-veg choices on her own will come naturally. Even so, most kids go through challenging phases and take on some strange eating habits from time to time throughout childhood. In this chapter, we talk about how to best handle those challenges.

For those parents who have recently adopted veganism and are introducing a new way of eating to your child, choosing veg foods on her own will likely be more challenging than for those families who were vegan from the start. In the following pages, we discuss ways to substitute vegan foods for animal-based products gradually, which gives your kids time to adapt.

Childhood is also the time they'll be introduced to all sorts of new junk foods, which can be quite exciting novelties. Remember the first time you saw cotton candy, foot-long licorice, or foot-long hot dogs at the ballpark? Banning all candy, fast food, and other junk foods from your child's diet may not be realistic. That said, you can minimize them without making her feel deprived, while still helping your child understand why junk foods should make up a tiny percentage of her food choices.

Finally, you learn the nuts and bolts nutritional needs of kids in this age group, and we encourage you to begin sharing these simple nutrition concepts with your child as young as 4 years old. Even preschoolers can begin to grasp some of the most basic ideas of why fruits and veggies, protein, carbohydrates, and natural fats are necessary to grow strong and healthy. You can teach them why it's important to limit or avoid processed foods, foods rich in unhealthy fats and sugar, and, of course, animal-based products.

Kids who understand what's good fuel for their bodies are laying the groundwork for developing a sense of mastery and control over what goes into their mouths. What a gift to give your child when they're this young, and what a foundation for her to continue to build upon throughout her life!

Nutrition Negotiation

"Pick your battles carefully," advised Dana's mother when we first began parenting. "But once you choose to enter into one, be sure you win." This sage advice may apply most directly to kids and food.

There are many times when entering a battle with your child over food is just plain wrong. "You must finish everything on your plate," is one of the oldest, most erroneous parent-child food fights. It causes your child to lose her ability to recognize hunger signals and know when she's actually hungry or full. This loss of hunger and *satiety* signals is a clear contributor to obesity.

Vegan Vocab

Knowing a sense of *satiety*—the state of being satisfied or physically full—is key to lifetime weight management. If children learn to eat even when full to "finish their plate," or eat for fun, out of boredom, or to soothe anxiety, it can lead to disordered eating and obesity.

Other times, food battles are futile. Expecting your child to eat a perfectly balanced diet every day, or believing that she will always forgo soda, candy, and treats throughout her entire childhood sets you both up to fail.

But from time to time, legitimate food battles must be fought— or at least negotiated. Parents need to find ways to guide children who consistently refuse to eat fruits, veggies, and whole grains onto a different path. To be healthy, all children must include those important food groups in their diets (or at least learn how to sneak them into food; see Chapter 9 for that) to some extent.

Parents also need to ensure their child is eating enough calories and nutrients, and practicing other basic self-care measures such as getting enough exercise and sleep. Guard your child's growth, health, behavior, mood, and ability to learn by setting up your home's food environment for the best choices possible, by being active in sports or other outdoor activities together, and by being aware of your child's sleep schedule.

Common Eating Challenges for Kids

In Chapter 3, we talked about strategies for working with the picky eater. Now let's dig further into other common kid eating quirks and offer some solutions. But first, be reminded: the best protection for a vegan child going through strange eating phases of any sort is including a daily multivitamin or fortified vegan foods in her daily diet, especially for vitamins B_{12} and D, as well as zinc, iron, riboflavin, DHA (docosahexaenoic acid), and calcium.

The following sections outline some common eating quirks and ways to quell them.

The Carb Queen

This child eats pasta, bread, crackers, rice, tortillas, and cereal in abundance but turns up her nose at nearly anything else—even anything on, in, or over those beloved carbs.

Solutions: Begin to put small amounts of healthful toppings, spreads, and vegetables on or in her favorite carb-based meals—and we mean *small* (barely noticeable) amounts: vegan Parmesan on the pasta, a few kernels of cooked frozen corn and carrots mixed into the rice, less than a spoonful of hummus on the tortilla. When you find a few that she'll eat, begin to add more of those. Then expand to other healthful additions such as tomato sauce on the pasta (again, *lightly* at first), small tofu chunks in the rice, or a couple bananas or strawberries cut in half on her cereal. Advance incrementally.

Because most carbs are rather blandly colored, color may be one of your child's hindrances, so first go with the simply colored fruits and veggies such as peeled apples, bananas, celery, corn—nothing outlandishly purple or, heaven forbid, green! Build up to those challenges.

Parent Trap

Simply do not introduce white bread to your child. The taste- and texture-stunting nature of bleached, white bread turns kids away from whole grains like nothing else. White bread is fortified, but the lack of natural nutrients and texture makes this a no-go food. It can be difficult to find whole-grain bread that doesn't contain dairy, so you might want to consider investing in a bread maker and making your own. Get your kids involved, too, if they're old enough.

Sugar Is King

Some kids want to eat dessert before, during, and after meals, but not just for the sweet taste. Anything with simple sugar gives them an immediate brain hit. They don't recognize it, but sugar can become like a mini-addiction for kids whose brains are sensitive to it. This is one of the trickiest vegan kid food issues to handle because so many great vegan desserts, candy, and treats are relatively healthful when compared with nonvegan desserts. But vegan sweets still must be consumed in moderation or limited for kids with sugar-sensitive brains.

Solutions: If your child has been a sugar hound for a while, you may need to retrain her taste buds by eliminating all foods containing simple, refined sugars for a while, until things like grapes and strawberries taste plenty sweet enough. Then, most candies, cookies, and even too much of a healthful sweet such as large portions of dried fruit or vegan brownies at breakfast seem unpalatable to them.

Vegan Voices

A great Halloween idea: When our child was two we made an orange paper Jack-o-Lantern and taped it to the door to signal "The Great Pumpkin" to come to our house .... The Great Pumpkin would trade out all the dairy products (overnight) for nondairy chocolate treats. The treats he left were homemade nondairy chocolates and other goodies.

—Kelly, Virginia

Even if you watch how much sugar and candy your child eats at home, she may be getting lots more than you would expect at school, scouting, after-school activities, even after sports practices. We've heard of teachers who toss marshmallows at students who answer math questions correctly!

It seems like kids are being "rewarded" with sugar everywhere these days. Help your kids learn self-control in these situations by simply telling them they can say, "No, thanks," or they can take a bite and throw the rest away. Educate them about the types of candy that aren't vegan, such as milk chocolate, caramels, marshmallows, and most baked goods.

If it's a more mild case of sugar love, consider compromise. For example, let her eat half of her slice of vegan cheesecake halfway through dinner (at least you know she's eating half of her healthful dinner!) and the other half afterward if she's still hungry (this helps her gauge her own hunger and gives less of a sugar rush by eating it in stages). Or provide dessert with lunch or dinner, but not both. Pair sugary snacks like raisins with a protein-rich food like peanut butter on celery to soften the sugar hit.

> **That's So Vegan**
>
> To learn more about carb and sugar cravings, as well as other food cravings, read the excellent book *Breaking the Food Seduction: The Hidden Reasons Behind Food Cravings—and 7 Steps to End Them Naturally* by Dr. Neal Barnard.

The sugar situation is a good opportunity to educate your child on the effects food can have on the brain and body. Even to a preschooler, you can say something as simple as, "If you eat this brownie at breakfast time, your body will feel hyper at first, then yucky, then tired. Too much sugar makes your brain get all garbled up, and it will be easier for you to get in trouble at school today. Sweets aren't breakfast food."

The Meal Skipper

Some kids go through phases when they really don't like to eat one particular meal of the day, typically breakfast or dinner. This eating glitch usually simply phases out after a while. But if it's ongoing for weeks at a time, you may want to replace the calories and nutrients lost from that meal in other ways.

Solutions: Keep your child at the table during family meals, even if she doesn't want to eat. The social aspect of family meals is still important, and many times your child will see something you're all eating that she likes and will nibble even if she was initially resistant to the full meal. Vegan energy bars are an excellent solution, especially at breakfast time. Kids who won't eat dinner will often want a snack before bed. Or they may wake up the next day and eat what seems like two or three breakfasts.

Be sure the snacks and breakfast foods you have at home are readily available and are the healthiest possible. Don't balk if your 10-year-old daughter eats two bowls of cereal, three veggie sausage links, and two bananas for breakfast if she didn't eat dinner the night before!

Meal Monotony

If your child gets stuck on eating cereal for breakfast, peanut butter and jelly for lunch, and veggie burgers for dinner for weeks, it's time to broaden her horizons. Sure, a multivitamin or fortified vegan food may make up for nutrients neglected by restricted food choices. But eating only limited foods over a long period of time can increase the possibility of nutritional deficiencies and may be a sign that she's developing disordered eating.

Solutions: Offer to prioritize her favorite meals she hasn't eaten for a while onto your weekly family dinner menu. Take her grocery shopping, and have her pick out a few new foods. Pack her school lunch with, yes, her standard PB&J, but also add a few surprises you know she's enjoyed in the past.

Don't become too rigid and expect your child to eat exactly what's prepared at every dinnertime for the family. This may be against the standard parenting advice to not become short-order cooks for your children, but if she's going through a phase with (or just naturally has) some real food aversions, we think accommodating your child with sides she likes, or allowing her to make her own portion of the main meal if she's old enough to make a sandwich, for example, shows your respect for her. In a vegan family, where great thought is usually given to the issue of respect for all beings with regard to food, consider that a child's preferences and aversions should be included in that respect.

Spice Isn't Nice

It's true, many kids do not like spicy or strongly flavored foods, including those containing onions and garlic. Spices are often a more grown-up preference, but that needn't be the case. Many spices are mild, such as mild yellow curry powder, cumin, and salt-free table spice blends, and some sweet herbs such as basil and rosemary make more economical, ethnic vegan dishes available for your family's weekly menu but also have very real health benefits. Rest assured, you can introduce new herbs and spices into your child's diet that will help ease them into spicy foods.

> **That's So Vegan**
>
> Plant an herb garden with your child. There's nothing more exciting for a child than to take ownership of a basil plant and then be able to pick some of it, smell it, put it in the pot, and watch it simmer in the tomato sauce. She'll notice—and take pride in—the flavor it adds to your meal.

Solutions: Start with the mildest form of spices possible. Serve spicy foods with coconut milk–based sauces, vegan cheese, or vegan sour cream, all of which help cool the palate. If your child finds the taste of foods containing garlic or onions too strong, consider roasting some garlic and having her try it spread on bread. Or have her use the garlic press to get used to the smell before eating it. Always sauté onions and garlic when serving to kids. Raw onions and garlic are simply too strong for most kids and may even upset their tummies.

Real Love for the Artificial

Some kids astoundingly, aggravatingly, absolutely love "fake" food and deplore the natural, homemade fare. Fresh, homemade applesauce? No way. Jarred applesauce with high-fructose corn syrup? Yum! Natural peanut butter? Yuk. Peanut butter full of oils, sugar, and salt? She'll eat it by the spoonful! The artificial colors and flavors of a powdered orange drink's fine, while the pulp in fresh squeezed orange juice is a turnoff for these antinaturals. What's a parent to do?

Solutions: If your child is older and her diet has included the less-healthful options for a while, the transition to natural foods will be a challenge for her taste buds. There are ways to ease her into preferring the better stuff. Consider blending the old choice with the newer, better version. For example, mix $^1/_4$ cup natural peanut butter with $^3/_4$ cup of the more processed kind she's used to. After a while, go $^1/_2$ and $^1/_2$, then $^3/_4$ to $^1/_4$, until she's switched with barely noticing.

Also, involve her in making some of the healthier options, like juicing fresh oranges with you. She's more likely to try it if she's made it. Use this as a nutrition teaching moment. Read the labels on the fake stuff, and ask her if she really wants to eat something she can't pronounce or has no clue what it is.

These common food challenges and the others our kids throw our way need not start a food fight. We can learn ways to respect their phases, guard their nutritional needs, and only pick the few battles we find absolutely necessary to win.

> **That's So Vegan**
>
> Read *A Consumer's Dictionary of Food Additives* (2009 edition) by Ruth Winter for a real eye-opener. Winter lists more than 12,000 food additives (some fine, some not) and explains how to read food labels so you really know what you're feeding your family.

Extra Challenge: Making the Transition for New Vegan Kids

Are you just starting the journey into veganism together with your children? Is your child becoming vegan due to the discovery of food allergies? Both situations have the extra challenge of transitioning taste buds from foods that are considered normal—dairy products, egg-based baked goods, or even meat—to the vegan alternatives.

Start with the foods she isn't closely attached to and switch them to foods that have the most comparable vegan substitutes. Then, add in the vegan foods that have distinct flavors but can be easily mixed or blended. For example, mix soy milk with cow's milk in equal parts and gradually continue to add more soy and less cow's until your child's transition to soy is complete.

Try to avoid calling animal product–based foods "real." For example, don't say, "We're using vegan mozzarella instead of real cheese on the pizza tonight." Instead, name the food's actual source: "cow's milk cheese" or "rice cheese." And even though "meat analog" is widely used in the veg community, it may sound rather foreign and unappealing to kids. Calling it a soy dog or a tofu sausage is much more likely to get a positive response from your child.

Basic Nutrition for Vegan Kids

Good news! According to the American Dietetic Association, vegan children's diets typically meet or exceed recommendations for most nutrients, and vegan kids eat more fiber and less total fat, saturated fat, and cholesterol than omnivorous kids.

Parents of vegan kids tend to be highly aware of nutritional issues. From the results of our survey, we believe vegan parents take a much greater interest in their children's food choices and overall nutrition than does the general parenting population.

That said, some nutrients need supplementation in vegan kids' diets, and parents should pay close attention to still other nutritional needs if their children are 100 percent vegan. Let's take a closer look at kids' nutritional needs. (For further discussion of nutrient and vitamin recommendations, see Chapter 9.)

Calories

This is the age when caloric needs begin to differ depending on your child's gender. Experts suggest a base daily calorie intake of about 1,200 calories for girls and 1,400 for boys ages 4 through 8. If your child is physically active—dancing, running, playing, swimming, perhaps participating in organized sports, etc.—those calorie needs increase.

If your child's diet is heavy in high-fiber foods, be extra sure to include foods rich in good fats like nuts, nut butters, and avocadoes, and encourage more snacking. Fiber may lead her to feel full faster, which can result in her eating fewer calories than necessary.

Protein

Protein recommendations for vegan children are 20 percent greater than those for omnivorous kids because plant proteins aren't digested as readily and plant amino acid quality is not as high as those from animal sources. Studies show most vegan kids' diets meet protein needs through soy and other plant sources without issue. Use a variety of plant-based protein sources such as tofu, beans, seitan, tempeh, nuts and seeds, nut butters, and soy-based meat analogs to ensure a variety of amino acids.

Vegan children ages 4 through 6 require about 26 to 28 grams plant-based protein per day. At age 7, protein needs generally increase to 31 to 34 grams per day due to children's increasing weight.

Vitamins

Vitamin D deficiency is a concern for all children because most don't spend enough time outdoors in the sun without sunscreen for appropriate vitamin D synthesis. There's a need to balance protection against sunburn and skin cancer with some sun exposure for vitamin D synthesis, which not only provides for strong bones but also myriad other functions in the body.

Vegan children don't drink vitamin D–fortified milk, so it's important that parents buy other products that are vitamin D fortified. Or vegan children should take a multivitamin that supplies vitamin D, as well as be exposed to at least 20 to 30 minutes of outdoor sunlight on skin that has not been covered with sunscreen two to three times a week. Vitamin D_2, which is plant-based, is just as effective as vitamin D_3, which is sourced from animal products.

> **That's So Vegan**
>
> The food choices at ballparks have come a long way in recent years. Check out PETA's Top 10 Vegetarian-Friendly Ballparks at www.peta.org/feat-veg-ballparks09.asp.

As we've discussed often in this book, vitamin B_{12} is an essential supplement for vegan kids because B_{12} is only found in animal-derived foods, and a prolonged deficiency can cause irreversible damage to the nervous system. Parents should also be sure their kids get enough riboflavin (vitamin B_2), either via a multivitamin or enriched foods.

Vitamin C is the darling of vitamins because it helps the immune system fight off illnesses of all kinds. Because of vegans' typically plentiful intake of fruits and veggies, vitamin C intake isn't an issue, but it's important to mention for vegan kids (especially those who are resistant to eating fresh fruits and vegetables, particularly citrus fruits) because of vitamin C's role in iron absorption.

Other vitamins to watch for are those in the B group and vitamin A.

Minerals

Zinc, iron, and especially calcium are important minerals to take note of in the diets of vegan children.

Calcium is essential for strong bones and teeth and the regulation of many other processes in the body. Studies have shown vegan children's diets to be low in calcium intake; however, relatively new calcium-fortified vegan products such as certain soy milk and orange juice brands are available now that make it easier for parents to meet their children's calcium needs. Signs of calcium deficiency include muscle spasms, dry skin and hair, brittle nails, and rarely, seizures. Vitamin D deficiency may be a sign of potential calcium deficiency.

Iron is essential for healthy blood production. Vegan children's diets have been found to contain iron levels above the recommended daily allowance.

Zinc, found most readily in meat, eggs, and nuts, is a very important nutrient for the body's insulin regulation and immune system. As discussed in Chapter 6, zinc acquired from plant sources may not be as bioavailable as animal-sourced zinc. Including in your child's diet foods high in zinc and protein such as nuts and legumes can enhance zinc absorption. A multivitamin containing zinc is also recommended.

Fats

Too much saturated fat, trans-fat, and cholesterol is not good for your child's health. The good news is, vegan diets are usually low in saturated fats, and cholesterol isn't a concern for the vegan diet because it's found only in animal products (and naturally produced in the human body).

Polyunsaturated fats, particularly omega-3 fatty acids, have been shown to promote good health and superior brain function from infancy through adulthood.

Currently the American Heart Association recommends total fat intake to be between 25 to 35 percent of calories. Most fats should come from sources of polyunsaturated and monounsaturated fatty acids, such as nuts, seeds, avocadoes, and healthy vegetable oils, like olive oil.

Algal oil is a veg alternative source of DHA that's added to dietary supplements or fortified foods such as soy milk. Vegan diets can include some ground flaxseed, canola oil, walnuts, and soy products. Care should be taken to watch omega-6 fatty acid intake. Omega-6s are fatty acids the body needs for healthy growth and development, but in too high of a concentration in the diet, they can lead to poor health through increased inflammatory responses. The omega-6 to omega-3 fatty acid ratio can be improved by reducing the use of oils such as corn oil and canola oil. The optimum ratio is 4:1, but vegan diets can be very high in omega-6s, even higher than red meat eaters.

If you're hoping your child will get enough omega-3 exclusively from flaxseed, walnuts, and soy, you may be wrong. Talk to your doctor about your child's particular needs and the most current recommendations, as research in this area is ongoing and rapidly developing. It may be essential to supplement up to 400 milligrams DHA from an algal source daily for proper development.

Sample Meal Plan for Vegan Kids

By the time your child reaches grade-school age, she will have developed a food personality all her own. This sample meal plan is simply a springboard for endless healthy vegan variations on your child's diet.

You've watched her grow and develop her unique food preferences, so now's the time to capitalize on all that groundwork and have some fun with the wide array of healthy veg foods and recipes you can continue to introduce to her!

Sample Meal Plan for Vegan Kids (4 to 8 Years)

Food Group	Number of Daily Servings
Grains	8 or more (A serving is 1 slice bread; ½ cup cooked cereal, grain, or pasta; ¾ cup ready-to-eat cereal.)
Protein foods	5 or more (A serving is ½ cup cooked beans, tofu*, tempeh, or TVP; 1 cup fortified soy milk*; 1 ounce meat analog; ¼ cup nuts or seeds*; 2 tablespoons nut or seed butter*.)

continues

Sample Meal Plan for Vegan Kids (4 to 8 Years)   (continued)

Food Group	Number of Daily Servings
Vegetables	4 or more (A serving is $\frac{1}{2}$ cup cooked or 1 cup raw vegetables*.)
Fruits	2 or more (A serving is $\frac{1}{2}$ cup canned fruit; $\frac{1}{2}$ cup juice*; or 1 medium fruit.)
Fats	2 or more (A serving is 1 teaspoon margarine or oil.)
Omega-3 fats	1 per day (A serving is 1 teaspoon flaxseed oil; 1 tablespoon canola or soybean oil; 1 table-spoon ground flaxseed; or $\frac{1}{4}$ cup walnuts.)
Starred food items	6 or more (A serving is $\frac{1}{2}$ cup calcium-set tofu; 1 cup calcium-fortified soy milk, orange juice, or soy yogurt; $\frac{1}{4}$ cup almonds; 2 table-spoons tahini or almond butter; 1 cup cooked or 2 cups raw broccoli, bok choy, collards, kale, or mustard greens.)

Reed Mangels, Ph.D., R.D., from "Simply Vegan," by The Vegetarian Resource Group; www.vrg.org.

Note: The starred servings also count as servings from the other groups at the same time. They aren't additional. The items in the Starred food items category are the foods you want your kid to consume because they're high in calcium. Serving sizes vary depending on the child's age.

The calorie content of the diet can be increased by greater amounts of nut butters, dried fruits, soy products, and other high-calorie foods.

A regular source of vitamin B_{12}–fortified nutritional yeast, vitamin B_{12}–fortified soy milk, vitamin B_{12}–fortified breakfast cereal, vitamin B_{12}–fortified meat analogs, or vitamin B_{12} supplements should be used.

The Least You Need to Know

- ◆ Prepare your child to begin making many of her own food choices by educating her about where foods come from and her nutritional needs.

- ◆ Pick your food battles, let many phases simply blow over, but insist that she meet her most important nutritional needs and find creative ways to help her do so. Even if your child isn't a naturally picky eater, kids often go through phases of strange eating habits.

- ◆ If your child aged 4 to 8 is just beginning to adopt a vegan diet, expect a time of transition. Start with the animal-based foods that are the least painful to give up or substitute with a plant-based alternative and ease into eliminating her animal-based favorites over time.

- ◆ Calcium, zinc, iron, vitamin B_{12}, and DHA are especially important to supplement in a vegan child's diet with a multivitamin and/ or enriched foods.

Chapter 8

Vegan Tweens (9 to 13 Years)

In This Chapter

- ◆ Growing like a tween
- ◆ What they watch impacts what they eat
- ◆ Tweens' increased nutrition needs
- ◆ A tween-appropriate meal plan

As your child progresses into the tween years, she'll begin to ask more sophisticated questions about everything—including your family's food choices. And she will likely point out any hypocrisies she notices in life—including yours.

On the flip side, as quickly as her hormones seem to change, a tween may change her mind about veganism like the wind changes direction, one day confident about your family's way of eating, the next day wondering if being different is worth the hassles. It's no wonder that one tween parenting book, Julie Ross's *How to Hug a Porcupine*, compares tweens to those quill-filled creatures. The myriad changes both boys and, even more acutely, girls begin to experience at this age add up to prickly moods, changing opinions, and skepticism about parents' ways of doing things.

In this chapter, we talk about what's happening to your tween's body at this stage and what you can do to nutritionally support those changes. You discover how your child's food choices are influenced by advertising and product placement and what you can do to counter that. As her parent, the balancing act of the tween years includes helping your child become confident in your family's way of eating and, at the same time, allowing her to question it and grow into her own views on veganism.

The Big Growth Spurt

Contrary to popular belief, the hormonal changes of puberty don't wait for the teen years. In fact, the female body begins to kick into hormone-changing gear as young as 7 or 8. So while the word *tween* may be a marketers' ploy to get younger kids to start acting—and buying—like teenagers, it can be a good term to help parents identify this unique stage of growth and development. Long before she hits 13 (many parents really begin to notice this around age 9 or 10), your child has already undergone some major physical changes that separate her from younger children, even though she's not yet a full-blown teenager.

That's So Vegan

Many studies of preadolescent lacto-ovo vegetarian girls suggest that being vegetarian may contribute to a delay in the onset of menstruation. This has health benefits, including decreased risk of breast cancer. Especially in light of the recent increase in girls going through puberty early for unknown environmental causes, this is more good news about being veg!

Healthy Body Image

In our body-conscious society, body image is an issue for both tween boys and girls, but especially girls. Studies show that by the time girls reach age 13, 80 percent of them report being dissatisfied with their body weight, and many have already been on diets.

The range for healthy weight gain of girls during puberty is 15 to 55 pounds, with a mean weight gain of 38.5 pounds. For boys, it's 15 to 65 pounds, with a mean weight gain of 52.2 pounds. Girls naturally have a 120 percent healthy increase in body fat during puberty, while boys drop body fat during the same time. This significant change in body type from boy to man and girl to woman can be particularly difficult for tween and teen girls to understand and embrace.

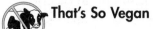 **That's So Vegan**

At least a few mainstream media outlets support girls with positive messages about body image. Check out *New Moon* magazine (www.newmoon.com) for girls ages 8 to 12 and also *American Girl* magazine (www.americangirl.com/fun/agmg).

According to the U.S. Department of Health and Human Services, young girls' body images are largely tied to their moms' attitudes about the subject. According to womenshealth.gov, these are some top reasons that may prompt young girls to have weight concerns:

◆ Having mothers concerned about their own weight.

◆ Having mothers who are overly concerned about their daughters' weight and looks.

◆ Natural weight gain and other body changes during puberty.

◆ Peer pressure to look a certain way.

◆ Struggles with self-esteem.

◆ Media images showing the ideal female body as thin.

Moms, be body confident! Focus on health, not weight. If you suspect your tween—girl or boy—has body image issues or is dieting, talk about it with them and their doctor. (For a more in-depth discussion about eating disorders, read Chapter 9.)

Media Pressures

Let's face it: most of your child's friends will likely eat fast food, candy, dairy, and meat. Not only will they be eating the foods you hope your child doesn't, but whenever they watch TV together, they'll be singing jingles about how much they love it. When your tween's friends are cooing at how cute the cows are in ads for foods that those very animals are confined or killed for, will she stand up for what she believes? This can be very confusing for vegan kids, especially tweens, who are constantly comparing their worldview about everything with those of their peers.

The numbers are astounding. Estimates show that American children see 18,000 to 30,000 ads every year. According to CommonSenseMedia.org, candy and snack foods account for 34 percent of ads targeted at kids, 28 percent are cereal ads, and 10 percent are peddling fast-food restaurants. Kids view an average of at least one food commercial *every 5 minutes* during Saturday morning cartoons. Most of those ads involve foods made with animal products, and virtually none are based on healthful, unprocessed foods like fruits and vegetables.

Some junk food products that happen to be vegan, such as Oreos, use advertising methods targeted at kids, too, including hiring sports figures popular with kids to promote their products. We venture to bet the tennis-star Williams sisters or the Manning brothers don't chow down on Oreos as part of their training diets even though they pitch the cookies in ads that clearly appeal to kids.

CommonSenseMedia.org offers these tips to keep your child's media diet as healthy as possible:

◆ Set limits on how much time your child spends with media, and stick to them.

◆ Keep the television, computer, and video game consoles out of your kids' bedrooms.

◆ Watch media with your kids, and point out when someone is selling them something that isn't good for them.

◆ Don't eat with the TV—your kids will look to your behavior as an example.

Parent Trap

Read more about how advertisers get inside the minds of kids in these books: *Consuming Kids: Protecting Our Children from the Onslaught of Marketing and Advertising* by Susan Linn; *Packaging Girlhood: Rescuing Our Daughters from Marketers' Schemes* by Sharon Lamb and Lyn Mikel Brown; and *Branded: The Buying and Selling of Teenagers* by Alissa Quart.

For vegan parents, we offer these extra ad-busting tips:

◆ If you can't beat 'em, join 'em. Some fruits and veggies now place cartoon characters and other kid-friendly celebs on their packages and stickers. If your child is more likely to eat a snack pack of baby carrots with Dora the Explorer on it, buy it.

◆ Explain the art of advertising to your child. Educate yourself about the types of advertising and the methods advertisers use to prompt food cravings in people and explain them to your child in kid-friendly language.

◆ Dive into veg-positive media. Petakids.com and others have fantastic vegan celeb promos, ads for vegan foods, and even vegan merchandise like T-shirts, backpacks, stickers, and bracelets your kids can use to promote their views on eating to the world.

◆ When you and your older child see a billboard, magazine ad, or television commercial that uses an animal to promote a food product made from that animal, write a letter together to the company to express your opinion.

This stage for the vegan child will be easier if her journey into being veg-confident began much earlier than the rocky tween years, when kids become rather uncertain about everything about themselves. If your family has been vegan for a while, your tween might surprise you with how confident, outspoken, and downright activist-ish she is in her beliefs about compassionate eating. If you've educated her on all the environmental, health, and animal benefits; served yummy vegan food at home; and as a result, she's seen the difference in her health and attitudes compared to meat eaters, veganism may be one of the few family beliefs she'll stand up for throughout these years.

Perhaps no matter when they began eating vegan, but especially if your family or child is new to veganism, be prepared to ride the roller coaster of tween change!

After she moves through tweenhood and reaches the older teen years, your child will settle into her own beliefs about eating animal-based products. Like any action or belief system, the more positive reasons you can establish for your child to follow what you've taught, the more likely she will be to choose to stay with—or come back to—that action or belief as an adult. The same holds true for food. In the tween years, the key words are *patience, positive guidance*, and *prepare for prickles!*

Basic Nutrition for Vegan Tweens

Tween nutritional and energy demands are equaled only by the infant year's demands, and you can help your child's nutritional needs meet these rapid growth spurts by learning the different needs of boys and girls during this time.

Other new differences come into play during the tween years, too:

◆ Whether your tween plays sports, what sport it is, how often, and for what duration

◆ Whether your daughter has started her monthly menstruation cycle (average age for American girls is 12)

◆ If your child has any attention, mood, or learning disorders that may be exacerbated by certain foods

◆ How her specific family genetics, ethnic background, and family's socioeconomic class is playing out in her years of puberty

Diving as deeply as necessary into these factors is beyond the scope of this book, so be sure to talk with your child's doctor if you have any concerns if your child's physical or mental health, growth, or lifestyle is particularly unique or worrisome in any of these areas.

Because age, weight, puberty stages, and gender difference result in such great variance during the tween years, talk to your child's doctor about her specific vitamin and mineral needs, too. Include some fortified foods in your tween's diet. Consider a high-quality multivitamin, or at the minimum a vitamin B_{12} supplement, for your tween.

The following sections outline some general nutritional needs of the 9 to 13 age group parents need to be aware of.

Calories

Female tweens need about 2,000 calories per day, and males need 2,300. This is the baseline, and the number increases as activity levels increase. No vegan tween should be on a calorie-restrictive diet.

To adults, this may seem like a high daily calorie intake, and tween girls who read women's fitness and beauty magazines may be misinformed about the number of calories a female their age should eat because they're comparing their needs to those of already-grown women. Encourage your vegan tween to eat well, eat often, and ignore information about dieting or proper weight maintenance from mainstream media sources that focus on women. It would be extremely rare for a mostly or all vegan tween or teen to be overweight unless their diet was based mainly on refined, processed vegan junk food.

Protein

Vegan tweens should consume about 40 grams of plant-based proteins per day. As with calories, this sounds like a lot of protein, but vegans need a few more grams of protein per day than meat eaters because of the reduced digestibility of plant-based proteins. This is more applicable for vegan children up to age 6 but still applies to a small extent for older vegan children. A Clif bar or a smoothie with veg protein powder, some nuts or nut butter, and one meal containing tofu or beans and brown rice would fulfill that need quite easily.

Tweens and teens need this much protein because their body is building mass faster than at any time since babyhood. Protein also helps the body rebuild stronger after athletics and helps the mind focus during studies.

This is not to say, however, that tween and teen boys, in particular, should be supported on using protein powders too often or in the place of whole foods. Moderation is key with all macro-nutrients, including protein.

Vitamins

Be sure good sources of vitamins A, C, and D, and the B-group vitamins are part of your vegan tween's diet. Hopefully by this time your tween's palate will have advanced to the point where she's willing to try a wide variety of plant-based proteins, fruits, and vegetables in varied and more complex combinations so you won't have to be as concerned overall as when she was younger and still more prone to food aversions.

Vegan tweens, however, still need at least a B_{12} supplement. Parents of girls, in particular, should strongly consider a calcium supplement for their tween daughters. For more specific suggestions, consult your tween's doctor or a registered dietician familiar with and supportive of vegan diets about supplement recommendations related to your child's unique health and diet profile.

Minerals

Calcium, iron, and zinc remain the most critical minerals to be aware of in the diet of vegan children, including tweens. Iron becomes even more important after girls begin menstruation.

If your tween is eating a varied diet based on whole, natural foods, these minerals should be easily acquired. Try to provide many fresh, colorful fruits and veggies, including dark leafy greens, as well as tofu and multigrain foods in their diet. Require a B_{12} supplement or B_{12}-fortified foods. Then all mineral needs should be met.

If your child is a picky eater into the tween years, a multivitamin may be necessary, as well as continued positive encouragement to try new foods. Talk to your child's doctor about her unique dietary profile related to mineral supplementation needs. Mineral supplementation should be done cautiously and with the recommendation of a physician or a registered dietician because mineral toxicity is possible.

Fats

About 25 to 30 percent of a tween's calories per day should come from healthy fat sources. (See Chapter 7 for more information on DHA requirements.) This is a critical time for parents to assist their tween in healthy fat intake because his growing, changing body needs fats and his body will crave fat. Choices and habitual behavior take front seat here. When his friends go to a fast-food restaurant, the vegan tween or teen is likely to choose french fries (bad fat) if his body is craving fat and healthy-fat foods haven't been part of his diet that day.

Healthy fats from plant-based sources include avocadoes, olives, olive oil, hummus made with tahini and olive oil, tofu, nuts, and nut butters. A DHA supplement can also provide some of the fat requirement and remove some of those fatty food cravings in some people. Healthy fats can be some of the most delicious, filling, diverse foods to incorporate into recipes and daily snacks. Just a handful of nuts a day in the backpack for a quick snack after school is a great start. Prepared properly and introduced often, your tween will easily meet their fat needs with these healthy choices instead of gravitating to unhealthy fats and getting into habits that can derail their diet into adulthood.

Sample Meal Plan for Vegan Tweens

Your tween's daily diet will vary greatly, depending on how active she is, whether she takes lunch to school or eats cafeteria-prepared lunches, how adventurous her palate has become, and how devoted you are as a family to sitting down for family meals. This sample menu plan offers a place to start with general requirements and basic ideas.

Sample Meal Plan for Vegan Tweens (9 to 13 Years)

Food Group	Number of Servings
Grains	10 or more (A serving is 1 slice bread; $\frac{1}{2}$ cup cooked cereal, grain, or pasta; $\frac{3}{4}$ cup ready-to-eat cereal.)

continues

Sample Meal Plan for Vegan Tweens (9 to 13 Years)   (continued)

Food Group	Number of Servings
Protein foods	6 or more (A serving is ½ cup cooked beans, tofu*, tempeh, or TVP; 1 cup fortified soy milk*; 1 ounce meat analog; ¼ cup nuts or seeds*; 2 tablespoons nut or seed butter*.)
Vegetables	4 or more (A serving is ½ cup cooked or 1 cup raw vegetables*.)
Fruits	2 or more (A serving is ½ cup canned fruit; ½ cup juice*; or 1 medium fruit.)
Fats	3 or more (A serving is 1 teaspoon margarine or oil.)
Omega-3 fats	1 per day (A serving is 1 teaspoon flaxseed oil; 1 tablespoon canola or soybean oil; 1 tablespoon ground flaxseed; ¼ cup walnuts.)
Starred food items	10 or more (A serving is ½ cup calcium-set tofu; 1 cup calcium-fortified soy milk, orange juice, or soy yogurt; ¼ cup almonds; 2 tablespoons tahini or almond butter; 1 cup cooked or 2 cups raw broccoli, bok choy, collards, kale, or mustard greens.)

Reed Mangels, Ph.D., R.D., from "Simply Vegan," by The Vegetarian Resource Group; www. vrg.org.

Note: The starred servings also count as servings from the other groups at the same time. They aren't additional. The items in the Starred food items category are the foods you want your tweens to consume because they're high in calcium. Serving sizes vary depending on the child's age.

The calorie content of the diet can be increased by greater amounts of nut butters, dried fruits, soy products, and other high-calorie foods.

A regular source of vitamin B_{12} like Vegetarian Support Formula nutritional yeast, vitamin B_{12}–fortified soy milk, vitamin B_{12}–fortified breakfast cereal, vitamin B_{12}–fortified meat analogs, or vitamin B_{12} supplements should be used.

The Least You Need to Know

- ◆ Be prepared. The hormonal and growth changes of puberty—and the moods that can go along with them—actually begin for kids at age 7 or 8 and are in full swing for many tween girls by age 12.

- ◆ Advertisers and the media try very hard to shape your child's eating habits, and usually not for the better. Be prepared to counter mainstream food ads with limits and a supplemental media diet of veg-positive media.

- ◆ A healthy body image is one of the greatest gifts you can give to your tween, especially your tween daughter.

- ◆ Your tween's nutritional requirements depend on many factors, including gender, activity level, and special needs. Go to your child's doctor with any questions or concerns specific to her situation.

Chapter 9

When Things Aren't Working

In This Chapter

- ◆ Signs your child needs something more
- ◆ Nutrition essentials
- ◆ Building a healthy relationship with health-care providers
- ◆ Different ways to the same goal

The medical literature is clear: carefully planned vegan diets are healthful for the majority of children. There are documented cases, however, of infants and children on 100 percent vegan diets who had severe deficiencies in important nutrients because of extreme picky eating, severe dietary limitations based on religious beliefs, a lack of basic nutritional knowledge on the part of the parents, or an eating disorder disguised as veganism. All these instances were avoidable.

In this chapter, we take a look at the signs of various nutritional deficiencies, list the nuts and bolts of bottom-line vegan nutrition for kids, and highlight some important sources of key nutrients, including both food sources and dietary supplements. If you and your child's physician have identified that she has a diet-related health issue, we discuss how to work with her doctor to correct course. And we tell you when, under certain circumstances, it may be necessary to back off of a 100 percent vegan diet for at least a time.

The vast majority of vegan parents are incredibly health conscious. By the very fact that you picked up this book, you're probably one of them. It's regrettable that the few vegan parents who haven't had the proper nutrition knowledge or have had other issues that led to their child's health problems have given veganism a bad name in some medical circles. That said, any parent—vegan or not—can have nutritional blind spots. This chapter helps bring those to light for us all.

Signs of Nutritional Deficiencies

No supporter of healthy vegan diets likes to hear about situations such as a vegan child who loses his vision due to a complete deficiency in vitamin A; a baby who becomes extremely ill due to his vegan breast-feeding mom's vitamin B_{12} deficiency; or a teen who says she's vegan and severely restricts her diet, but really has an underlying serious eating disorder.

Unfortunately, these situations have happened and could happen again unless vegan parents have the right nutrition information, healthy dietary practices, common sense, and sound reasons for raising a vegan child.

Even if nutrient deficits aren't as extreme as these examples, many children in industrialized nations aren't getting optimal nutrition, vegan or otherwise. Even the belief that people—vegan or omnivorous—can get all the nutrients they need for optimal health from food alone is hotly debated in the medical community. Some experts suggest it's no longer possible to meet full nutrient needs without a multivitamin and mineral supplement and other supplements like DHA because of poor soil quality, genetic engineering, storage and transport of food over long distances, and increased environmental toxins.

Many of the calories children consume today are empty calories, devoid of whole-food nutrients. Kids who don't eat adequate protein or who lack healthy fats, like DHA, often have a difficult time staying focused in school. Most of these mild deficiencies would not register on a blood test, but they show in the child's behavior, general health, and wellness.

Several low-grade deficiencies may sneak into American families' everyday lives. It's estimated that almost all Americans are at least somewhat deficient in vitamin D. Educating women of child-bearing age about optimal levels of folic acid in their diets to prevent birth defects is an important health concern in our society. With the many challenges the *SAD* (*standard American diet*) presents, parents need to learn everything we can about basic childhood nutrition to protect our children against some of the most avoidable health-related problems.

In this section, we'll review the nutritional needs vegan parents must be most aware of to ensure healthful diets for our children. Read on for signs of significant nutritional deficiencies, as well as good food sources of these nutrients. If you suspect any of these deficiencies in your child, it is important to consult with your child's primary care physician.

> **Vegan Vocab**
>
> **SAD,** or the **standard American diet,** is the sugar- and meat-heavy diet typical of Westernized populations and quickly spreading throughout the globe. Many health problems, such as obesity, diabetes, certain cancers, and heart disease have been associated with the SAD.

Iron

Physical symptoms of iron deficiency include pale skin, lack of energy, pale lower lids of the eye, shortness of breath with exercise, or a fast heart beat.

Good kid-friendly food sources of iron include the following:

◆ Beans

◆ Blackstrap molasses

◆ Bran flakes

◆ Enriched grain products

- Pumpkin seeds
- Tofu

Eating food cooked in a cast-iron skillet also increases iron absorption. If you give your child an iron supplement, give her orange juice to drink at the same time because vitamin C increases iron absorption. (Be sure to keep supplements containing iron out of reach of your child and in a childproof container.)

Vitamin D

Vitamin D deficiency can lead to weak bones, and some researchers suggest it may be related to cancer, muscle aches, and neurological problems. Symptoms of a vitamin D deficiency include general weakness and muscle aches.

Good sources of vitamin D include fortified foods like vitamin D–fortified soy milk, as well as moderate sun exposure to the hands and face 2 or 3 times a week for 20 to 30 minutes for light-skinned children.

Vegan Voices

We cannot endorse or recommend any particular brand of supplement, but some vegan parents we surveyed mentioned these vegan and nonvegan vitamin brands as their family's vitamin choice: Multigenics, Higher Nature, Animal Parade, Nature's Plus, Rainbow Light, Trader Joe's, and VegLife's Vegan Kids. Most parents mentioned B_{12} as the main reason they provided a multivitamin for their children.

Zinc

Zinc deficiency is characterized by decreased taste, rough skin, inability of the eyes to react to changes in light, memory loss, and learning problems. In severe cases, hair loss, tremors, and weight problems have also been reported.

Good food sources of zinc include the following:

- Bran flakes
- Fortified breakfast cereals

- Lentils

- Tahini

- Textured vegetable protein (dry flakes made from soy flour that are rehydrated and used in many recipes such as chili or tacos as a meat substitute)

Vitamin B$_{12}$

Severe B$_{12}$ deficiencies can cause irreversible neurological damage and must be safeguarded against in vegan children's diets with a dietary supplement and/or fortified foods. Mild to moderate B$_{12}$ deficiency is characterized by fatigue, loss of appetite, and nausea. Severe B$_{12}$ deficiency causes anemia; numbness and tingling of arms and legs; recurrent upper respiratory infections; and other strange symptoms like sore tongue, paranoia, and nervousness.

Good sources of B$_{12}$ are limited in the vegan diet. A vitamin supplement is the best way to ensure proper B$_{12}$ intake in vegan children. Fortified foods like breakfast cereals, meat analogs, and nutritional yeast often contain B$_{12}$.

Calcium

Calcium deficiency isn't a condition generally noted in children by the mainstream medical community. A lack of meeting calcium needs in childhood, however, is a contributor to long-term bone health because the largest calcium stores are laid in the bones during the formative years. The American Dietetic Association states, "limited data suggest that calcium intakes of vegan children are below current recommendations."

Good kid-friendly sources of calcium include the following:

- Blackstrap molasses

- Calcium-fortified orange juice

- Soy milk

- Tofu

Avoid caffeine in your child's diet, not only because it can affect her behavior but also because caffeine contributes to calcium loss. It may be a minimal amount of calcium loss, but when many vegan kids' calcium intake is already marginal, any loss is too much.

Vitamin A

Vitamin A deficiencies are rare but can lead to blindness and can be life-threatening. (There is also such a thing as too much vitamin A, which causes toxicity and myriad symptoms including nausea, vomiting, and clumsiness.) A vegan diet is not likely to be deficient in vitamin A as long as your child regularly eats multicolored vegetables. If your vegan child is an extremely picky eater or completely avoids vegetables, she could become vitamin A deficient. Supplement with a standard multivitamin.

Good kid-friendly sources of vitamin A are these:

◆ Apricots

◆ Carrots

◆ Mangoes

◆ Watermelon

Parent Trap

More isn't always better when it comes to vitamin and mineral supplements. There is a possibility of overdose or toxicity at higher-than-recommended levels. Unless otherwise advised by your child's doctor, stick with a regular daily child's multivitamin that does not exceed the standard FDA recommendations and a DHA supplement.

Protein

Studies suggest that vegan kids get as much or more protein than nonvegan kids. A severe protein or amino acid deficiency is called kwashiorkor and is rarely seen in developed countries. Typically, it's found in newly weaned children in developing countries whose diets are primarily based on corn, rice, and beans. Signs of kwashiorkor include lethargy, apathy, redness in skin and skin peeling, and sparse and thin hair and nails. Another protein deficiency disease, marasmus, is characterized by weight loss; listlessness; wrinkled, loose skin; and frequent small stools with mucus.

Bottom line: vegan kids in industrialized countries are no more likely to have a protein deficiency than omnivorous kids. Kids at risk of protein deficiencies are those whose parents are severely impoverished or who follow fad diets.

Good vegan sources of protein include these:

◆ Meat analogs

◆ Nuts and nut butters

◆ Seeds

◆ Tofu and other soy products

Avoid using rice milk exclusively for your kids' main drink. It's the poorest protein source among plant-based milk options.

DHA/Omega-3

There are few outward signs of omega-3 fatty acid/DHA deficiency. A lack of DHA may contribute to poor retinal development in infancy. Long-term health problems such as cancers and memory and mood disorders are associated with all omega-3 deficiencies, not just DHA. In kids, dry skin, behavioral problems, learning delays, and recurrent illness such as respiratory infections and colds can signal a deficiency in omega-3s. Omega-3s, including DHA, are essential to the overall health and well-being of you and your child.

Good sources of omega-3s are these:

◆ Flaxseeds

◆ Olive oil

◆ Walnuts

That's So Vegan

Vegan algae-sourced DHA brands for kids include Solaray, Deva, Thorne, VegLife, Dr. Fuhrman's DHA Purity, and Source Naturals.

That said, those sources of omega-3s are not as optimal as DHA and need to be limited to ensure a proper ratio of omega-3s in your child's diet (see Chapter 4). Only fish and algae-sourced supplements are direct sources of DHA. Many child behavior experts now recommend providing all children with a DHA supplement.

Calories

When a child has a deficiency of calories in her diet, it will show up as a low BMI (body mass index) for her age. (Find an online BMI calculator website in Appendix B.) Kids who aren't consuming enough calories will also have low energy, dry skin, irritability, delayed puberty, and poor attention.

Good sources of calories include the following:

♦ Avocadoes

♦ Bananas

♦ Meat analogs

♦ Nuts and nut butters

♦ Potatoes

♦ Soy and nut milks

♦ Whole grains

Bottom-Line Nutrition

Keeping track of how much vitamins, minerals, and other nutrients your vegan child needs at various ages and stages of development can be complicated and sometimes confusing. To help sort it all out, use the following handy table to view at a glance all the recommended daily allowances for nutrients especially important in the diets of vegan children.

Important Recommended Daily Nutrients

Nutrient	Supplement Dose	Foods
B_{12}	Toddlers (1 to 3 years): RDA 0.9 mcg/day; kids (4 to 8): RDA 1.2 mcg/day; tweens (9 to 13): RDA 1.8 mcg/day; teens (14 and up): RDA 2.4 mcg/day; pregnant women: RDA 2.6 mcg/day; nursing moms: RDA 2.8 mcg/day	Fortified cereals, nutritional yeast, or other fortified foods; all other sources are animal based.
Zinc	Infants (0 to 6 months): 2 mg/day; infants and toddlers (7 months to 3 years): 3 mg/day; kids (4 to 8): 5 mg/day; tweens (9 to 13): 8 mg/day; teen girls (14 to 18): 9 mg/day; teen boys (14 to 18): 11 mg/day	Peanuts, beans, whole-grain cereals, brown rice, and whole-wheat bread. Pumpkin seeds offer one of the most concentrated nonmeat food sources of zinc.
Calcium	Toddlers (1 to 3): 500 mg/day; kids (4 to 8): 800 mg/day; tweens and teens (9 to 18): 1,300 mg/day	Calcium-fortified soy milk and juice, calcium-set tofu, soybeans, soy nuts, bok choy, broccoli, collards, Chinese cabbage, kale, mustard greens, and okra. 4 ounces firm tofu or $\frac{3}{4}$ cup collard greens contain as much or more calcium as 1 cup cow's milk.
Vitamin D	The Academy of Pediatrics increased the recommended minimum daily intake of vitamin D to 400 IU daily for all infants and children, including adolescents.	Very few vegan foods contain vitamin D. Mushrooms, when exposed to the sun, can be good sources of vitamin D.

Parent Trap

A note about raw diets: according to the American Dietetic
Association and Dieticians of Canada, fruitarian and completely
raw diets cannot be recommended for infants and children because they
have been associated with impaired growth. Kids should enjoy many
healthy raw foods along with cooked foods as part of an overall balanced vegan diet.

Working With Your Health-Care Provider

If something isn't working in your child's diet or she otherwise just
isn't up to her usual state of health, see her doctor as soon as possible.
Hopefully, you've established a good relationship with your health-care
provider (see Chapter 6 for tips on that) and he or she will be ready to
work with you knowing your child's health history and your family's
dietary choices.

If you don't have an established health-care provider and your
child has a suspected diet-related health problem, it's a roll of the dice
what kind of reaction you'll get when you tell a physician new to your
family that your child's vegan. Try to find a veg-friendly physician by
word of mouth, either through other vegan families, your local health
food store, or by calling clinics and asking some questions.

Most importantly, *don't lie about your child's diet*. A complete health
history gives the doctor important clues into what's going on so the
problem can be identified and solved.

Clinically, the doctor will most likely want you to provide a general diet history and will take your child's height and weight and plot it
into a general growth chart. If you're working with a new doctor and
have information on your child's height and weight from other medical visits in previous years or even from a home scale, bring that along,
too. Based on symptoms, the doctor may order blood tests to measure
any of the nutritional deficiencies mentioned in this chapter. When the
blood test results come back in about 2 or 3 days, the physician will be
able to direct you in what can be done to correct course.

Enlisting the help of a dietician may be helpful if your child has a particularly stubborn diet-related health issue. Find a dietician in your area by logging on to www.eatright.org and clicking on "Find a Nutrition Professional."

Other Means of Support

Here are some other daily lifestyle choices you can make to further support your child's optimal health:

- Be sure she gets enough sleep.
- Include regular opportunities for exercise in her day.
- Provide a daily multivitamin/mineral supplement and a DHA supplement.
- Teach her stress management through activities like kids' yoga, family meal times, parent-child outings, spending time in nature, and connecting to your chosen faith community.
- Promote learning (rather than grades) in school.
- Don't overschedule. Let your child be a kid!

When It's Time to Consider Other Options

You may need to consider that a 100 percent vegan diet may not be right for your child at the present time if …

- Your child has significant food allergies or sensitivities to foods that make up a large portion of the vegan diet such as soy, beans, nuts, or gluten.
- Your child has been diagnosed with an eating disorder such as anorexia and is advised by her doctor to expand her food choices.
- After multiple efforts on your part to expand her dietary choices, your child still limits her diet to a small number of foods due to extreme picky eating and will eat few fruits and vegetables.

- Your child has fallen off her growth curve, and your attempts to alter her vegan diet to increase calorie, fat, and food intake hasn't helped her weight gain to resume to a normal level.

- She's very resistant to the idea of eating 100 percent vegan and has expressed ongoing and adamant opposition to being labeled vegan by her friends.

If a child has a nutritional deficiency or other ongoing complication related to her diet, as her parents, you must set aside black-and-white, purist ideals. When health and weight issues become paramount, *the most important thing is that the child is fed.* You need not feel guilty for not meeting your goals perfectly for your child's diet. No matter what other foods must be included, you can still find ways to incorporate many healthy plant-based foods into her diet.

It's important to meet your child where she is today, and you can revisit the issue of veganism at a later time.

The Least You Need to Know

- Even if nutrient deficits aren't extreme, many children aren't getting optimal nutrition, vegan or otherwise. Many of the calories children consume today are empty, devoid of whole-food nutrients.

- A daily multivitamin and mineral supplement plus a DHA supplement are simple ways to protect against nutritional deficiencies.

- It's important to stay up to date on your child's changing nutrition needs as they grow because many vitamin, mineral, and macronutrient recommendations change significantly with each stage.

- Work closely and honestly with a health-care provider when a nutritional deficiency or other health issue in your child is suspected.

Part 3

Stocking the Vegan Kitchen

A vegan kitchen—and a kid-friendly one at that!—is easy to set up once you get to know some essential components such as healthful, kid-friendly pantry staples; meat, egg, and dairy substitutes; and made-for-kids kitchen tools. A few fun, easy, and healthful adaptations can make the difference between creating kid-pleasing meals or family flops.

Like all kids, most vegan kids love helping out in the kitchen and trying fun new foods *if* you serve them the good stuff. Stock your kitchen right, get them involved in the preparation process, and serve kid-friendly meals, and feeding your vegan children will be infinitely easier.

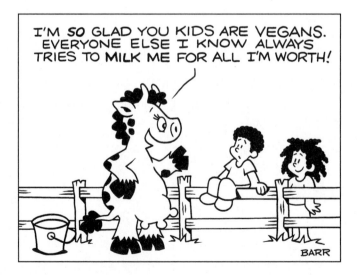

Chapter **10**

Let's Go Shopping!

In This Chapter

- ◆ Making grocery shopping stress free—it *is* possible!
- ◆ Time- and money-saving shopping tips
- ◆ Stocking your vegan pantry
- ◆ Vegan-friendly food allies

For busy parents, grocery shopping is a chore, at best. For busy vegan parents, the added frustration of constantly searching for specialty products and methodically reading fine print for hidden animal ingredients, all while their child is trying to escape from the shopping cart, can become a weekly test of anger management.

For vegan kids, the overstimulation of stores filled with animal products is both enticing and disheartening. Most kids will ask, "Why can't I have …?" and parents need to be patient and explain. If the meat department cannot be avoided, kids' questions often change from personal wants to "What's that bloody-looking red stuff in that case?" and "Why are those lobsters in that tiny tank?" Parents need to be honest and explain.

If your weekly grocery run feels more like going to the guillotine than grabbing the family grub, this chapter's for you. We show you how to make grocery shopping smooth, efficient, and fun—even when you have to bring your little shopper(s) along. Like most good things in life, though, eating vegan and healthy doesn't come cheap. We share ways to minimize the costs while maximizing flavor and nutrition for your vegan child. Finally, we talk about strategies to lower your monthly grocery bill and include some of our favorite frugal vegan meals.

So what exactly does a kid-friendly vegan grocery cart include? This chapter highlights the essentials of the vegan family pantry and fridge. Most items we suggest can be found in any moderate- to well-stocked grocery store, but some will likely take a (worthwhile) trip to your local health food or natural foods store.

After reading this chapter, finding healthy vegan food for your family will become a pleasure.

Stress-Free Family Grocery Shopping

Take a nearly empty pantry, add one time-crunched parent in a grocery store with no list or meal plan in hand, sprinkle in a hungry kid or two, and you have the recipe for a stressful, expensive shopping trip. It takes time to organize a list to be sure you have all necessary ingredients at home for enough meals for the week. Adding the vegan twist usually means some of those items may not be readily available in your local grocery store and will require another stop or two. Poorly planned shoppers often bring home a lot of snacks and desserts but only a couple of complete, healthful meals.

The saying, "An ounce of prevention is worth a pound of cure," fits the vegan grocery bill. Take some time up front to organize your kitchen and your family's favorite meal plans. Then search out which stores have what you need at the best prices and develop a meal plan/grocery system that works best for your family. Your budget will stretch farther, your patience will be stretched less, and your belt is less likely to need stretching due to unhealthy food impulse buys. Most importantly, you and your child are more likely to eat healthier with less stress.

Time Savers

The following time savers help you breeze through the vegan food gathering process. You might be surprised at how pain-free shopping can become. Yes, some of these do require more than a couple minutes up front, but you'll consistently save time every week after they're done once every year or so.

Organize Your Pantry

First things first, put all your dried and canned goods in order (tomato sauces, pastes, etc.; canned vegetables; jarred nut butters; oils and vinegars; spices; etc.) and keep them organized so it's easy to see what you're missing. If you're short on pantry space, a stand-alone metal pantry rack that can be stored in a broom closet or in the corner of your kitchen is an affordable alternative.

Make Your Lists (and Check Them Twice ...)

Now, with your pantry organized, make a list of all regularly needed pantry and fridge items and post it on the inside of the pantry door and the side of the fridge so you can check what you need.

Next, keep a simple date notebook of meals your family enjoyed and rotate them (trying some new experiments every now and again) to create weekly menus before you shop. Add new recipes into the notebook for a quick ingredients check.

Before you head to the store, be sure you have your list. Find a printable grocery list online, or use what's included with your computer's software (Microsoft Word has a reasonably good one). Simply delete the animal products included, and add your vegan staples to it.

Create a System

Decide what frequency and time of day works best for your family, figure out when your favorite stores are least crowded and most stocked, and stick to that info. For some families, that means multiple small trips each week. For others, monthly cart-fillers. For the rest of us, something in between.

Much depends on the size of your family, the ages of your kids, and your work schedule. What's most important is that you experiment to figure out when the time is right for you to keep your pantry stocked with healthful vegan fare so no one is settling for BPOs (best possible options) too often, and so the experience is more nourishing than exhausting.

When you've decided on your system, do a run by yourself every now and again. Once kids are mobile, it's next to impossible to keep an eye on them and read every label and monitor price comparisons as closely as you need to be a frugal vegan shopper. Do yourself and your budget a favor, and ask your parenting partner to watch the kids or get a sitter and make a grocery run all by yourself every month or two.

> **Parent Trap** _____
>
> Myriad hidden animal ingredients are in food you might not have thought of. Top offenders include gelatin, lecithin (not soy-based), rennet, and casein. For an extensive list of hidden animal products check out www.caringconsumer.com/resources_ingredients_list.asp. For kid-friendly, brand-name foods that are surprisingly vegan, see www.petakids.com/accvegan.html.

When you do take the kids, take your parenting partner, too, and split up the list. Meet at the checkout in half the time. (A race to the finish may not be a bad idea!)

Prep the Kiddos

If you have to tote them along to the store, be sure your kids are well rested, well fed, and recently pottied before heading out. The after-school/after-work grocery run is *the* top time to avoid. Kids are hungry, everyone's tired, and no one's had a chance to decompress before walking into an enclosed building full of sight, sound, and scent stimulation. Not a good combination for stressed families!

If you must go at this time, be sure you stash a bag of healthy bars, nuts, or vegan snack mix (see Chapter 15) in your car to munch on before you go in or even while you shop.

Money Savers

Groceries consume a major chunk of most families' monthly budgets. Eating vegan, choosing some or all organics, and providing your child with some of the fun snack foods and desserts he loves can add up quickly.

The following sections offer some money-saving tips to help you fill your cart without draining your wallet.

Shop Smart

Most frugal shopping experts recommend this simple trick, and it applies to vegan families as well: reduce the number of purchases you make from the center aisles where the most processed, packaged, and expensive foods are placed.

If you've gone through the time saver of making a list, as recommended earlier in this chapter, use it to avoid impulse buys.

Stores are always removing slow-moving items from their shelves. Check these racks and bins for items that are on their way out of the store and into your home.

Buy In Bulk

Many health/natural food stores allow regular customers to order items in bulk and pay less. Turn grocery store sales into your own bulk order, and buy as many as you can afford up to their offer limit. Consider buying a membership to one of the big-box wholesale club stores. They don't intentionally cater to the veg crowd, but they do carry many kid-friendly staple items like pastas, oils, salad dressings, and big bags of root veggies that can add up to substantial savings over time.

This goes for frozen items, too. Many freezer-friendly veg products such as meat substitutes, potato products, frozen ice-cream alternatives, premade vegan kids' and adults' meals, frozen fruits for smoothies, and frozen veggies have long freezer lives. Stock up during sales.

Buy Produce In-Season, Local, and Organic

Veggies in season are almost always cheaper. Fruits from a farm in your home state will be much cheaper (and potentially more likely organic) than those flown in from Spain.

Also, consider buying organic when you can. According to the Environmental Working Group's *Shopper's Guide to Pesticides*, the fruits and vegetables with the worst pesticide coverage are, in this order: peaches, apples, bell peppers, celery, nectarines, strawberries, cherries, kale, lettuce, grapes (imported), carrots, and pears. If you can, buy these in organic forms. The foods with the lowest use of pesticides are onions, avocados, sweet corn, pineapples, mangoes, asparagus, sweet peas, kiwi, cabbages, eggplants, papayas, watermelons, broccoli, tomatoes, and sweet potatoes.

Do It Yourself

Before you toss premade vegan foods and snacks in your shopping cart, think about what you can substitute or make at home for less dough.

For example, make simple home fries rather than buying frozen french fries. Veggie burgers and other *meat analogs* can get expensive. Homemade lentil burgers that you can make, freeze, and heat up are more economical—and contain no additives. If you have a garden, homemade salsa from your own tomatoes will likely be much cheaper than the store-bought kind.

Vegan Vocab

Vegan families vary widely on how much they consume **meat analogs**—plant-based foods that closely resemble animal-based counterparts—such as veggie bacon, burgers, sausages, and hot dogs. Typically soy-based, most are highly processed and some brands, including most Morningstar Farms products, contain milk or eggs. On the upside, truly vegan meat analogs offer a great animal-free way for kids to eat usually meat-based socially mainstream foods.

Check Prices and Coupons

Don't assume prices will be better on some items in one store than the other. Health food stores may be cheaper on some staples, and mainstream grocers may have better prices on some health specialty items. Keep a little pocket notebook with you to record prices, and you won't be fooled.

Most coupons in mainstream Sunday newspapers or coupon websites don't apply to vegan foods. But many health food stores' own coupon books contain great deals on vegan-relevant staples. And the websites of vegan food companies often have great coupons you can use at any store.

> **That's So Vegan**
>
> Check around online to find sites that offer coupons and other specials. Here are some good places to start: Silk (www.silksoymilk. com/specialoffers.aspx), Rice Dream and others (www.tastethedream. com), Tofurkey (www.tofurky.com), and WildWood Organics (www. pulmuonewildwood.com/promo.asp).

Pick Your Splurges

What items can you skimp on, and what can't be compromised? In our Italian home, quality canned and jarred tomato products are a must. The cheaper brands taste too acidic. On busy weeks, you may choose to splurge for the premade hummus and a few night's worth of premade frozen vegan meals, but forgo prepackaged snacks like crackers, cookies, and ice cream and instead provide your kids fruits and veggies and peanut butter at snack time.

Some vegan kid favorites are maple syrup, tahini, vegan ice-cream treats, and premade vegan kids' meals, but these can be quite expensive. If you do buy these items, space them out so you don't need to buy all of them in the same week or month. Watch for sales and stock up.

Eat Ethnic

Some of the most affordable vegan meals are traditional ethnic dishes that are meat-free, kid-friendly, and full of flavor and protein—and made with just a few, affordable ingredients. Learn how to prepare foods from India, the Caribbean, Mexico, the Middle East, and Africa to save money on your grocery bill and expand your child's culinary palate.

In our survey, parents listed these affordable meals most often as their kids' favorites: vegan pizza, rice and lentils, veg soups and chili, hummus and pitas, rice and beans, bean burritos, veg tacos, scrambled tofu, and vegan macaroni and cheese. These meals fill the tummy without breaking the bank!

Shopping with Kids: Sanity Savers

When you choose—or have no choice but—to bring the kids along, you can increase your chances of everyone coming out of the grocery store still speaking to each other with a few creative guidelines.

Grocery shopping can be a fun learning experience when the entire family goes together. Kids learn natural lessons about budgeting, price comparison, checking for animal products in foods, and the art of carrying out an organized list.

The Insta-Treat

Don't wait to give your child a treat for good behavior at the end of the trip. Offer one up front, and you set the expectation that you know they will cooperate. (If they don't, the treat can always be put back at the checkout aisle or saved for later.)

The insta-treat provides the added bonus for vegan kids of choosing treats from the first section of the store, usually the produce section, rather than waiting for the checkout aisle treats such as candy bars, gum, and chips. It encourages kids to choose healthy treats like cut fruit in bowls, a bag of grapes, or one of the many delicious bottled smoothies often stocked in produce sections. And it shows them you aren't waiting to see if they're going to be cooperative. It's simply expected.

That's So Vegan

Parents, put in a call, letter, or comment card to your favorite grocery store's managers encouraging them to stock fruits, veggies, smoothies, and other healthy treats instead of candy, gum, soda, and tabloids in checkout lines. Many stores now have "family lane" checkout aisles that drop the bad stuff. But few have replaced it with the good. Push them to take the next step.

Think Comfort

Grocery stores can be difficult, overstimulating places for many kids, so make it as physically comfortable as possible. Babies and toddlers may need a cart cover to soften the seat. Kids of all ages may need a jacket or sweater, especially because veg families spend a lot of time shopping in the colder sections of stores where the fresh produce and frozen foods are located.

If your child has sensory integration issues, grocery stores may be a difficult place for them. You may need to limit trips to smaller health food store runs.

Here's a good place to mention the preshopping bathroom run again! If your child isn't feeling well, do everything possible to keep them home during grocery trips. The sights and smells can quickly overwhelm them.

Enlist Help

Matching appropriate jobs to his age but starting as young as 3, your child can help take nonbreakable items from shelves and place them into the cart, check prices, and even push a younger sibling in a stroller. When he can read well, he becomes a big help by reading items on your shopping list to you and checking them off.

At the checkout counter, keep everyone busy emptying the cart.

Keep It Fun

Get excited when something you like is finally in season and ripe.
Comment on colors, flavors, and textures of fruits and veggies, and
other healthful food qualities throughout the store. Teach your child
how to smell if a mango's ripe or how to thump a melon. Avoid walking
through the meat section.

Dance to the bad Muzak. Let your kids know how grateful you
are for the bountiful supply of healthful, vegan food to which your
family has access, whether your budget currently allows for the bare
essentials, gourmet fare, or somewhere in between.

Stocking the Kid-Friendly Pantry

Good meals start with the basics. A pantry stocked with kid-friendly
vegan staples makes it easier to whip up a last-minute dinner that will
please everyone in the family. A kid-friendly pantry is also much more
likely to be a frugal pantry because you don't need to produce gourmet
fare to impress kids.

Here are some of our favorite veg-friendly brands:

- Amy's Kitchen
- Annie's Naturals
- Boca
- Bragg's
- Earth Balance
- Eat in the Raw Parma!
- Eden
- Ener-G
- Frieda's
- LightLife
- Orgran
- Pacific Natural Foods
- Rice Dream
- Silk
- Soy Delicious
- Tofurkey
- Tofutti
- WildWood
- Willow Run
- Yves

The following basic lists of pantry staples set the stage for kid- and crowd-pleasing meals. Many of the items listed are necessary for the recipes found in this book. Obviously, there are thousands of other fruits, veggies, beans, and grains to enjoy. And the great vegan specialty products such as marshmallows, soy whipped cream, and vegan tuna may be something for your family to try according to your child's tastes and adventure level. The foods listed here are simply what we consider the "kid-friendly basics" and a great start to show vegan diets for kids are far from restrictive!

> **That's So Vegan**
>
> Every attempt has been made to ensure the foods on this list are vegan, but we concur with what PETA posts on its vegan food list online: "Boycotting products that are 99.9 percent vegan sends manufacturers the message that there is no market for that particular food, which ends up hurting more animals."

Meat Analogs

From chicken nuggets to barbecue ribs, you can find kids' favorite meat-substitute products in abundance at most well-stocked grocery stores.

- ❑ Barbecue ribs
- ❑ Breakfast sausage links
- ❑ Burger crumbles
- ❑ Chick nuggets
- ❑ Chick patties
- ❑ Chick strips
- ❑ Italian sausages
- ❑ Lunch meats
- ❑ Marinated *tofu* cutlets
- ❑ Plain tofu

- ❑ Seitan (many varieties)
- ❑ Tempeh (many varieties)
- ❑ Tofu turkey
- ❑ Veggie bacon
- ❑ Veggie beef strips
- ❑ Veggie burgers
- ❑ Veggie chorizo
- ❑ Veggie hot dogs
- ❑ Veggie pepperoni

Vegan Vocab

Tofu is a soybean curd food that originated in China. To make it, soybeans are soaked in water, with a small amount of magnesium chloride, and formed into blocks. Just 3 ounces tofu supplies 14 grams protein and 10 percent of an adult's daily iron needs.

Nondairy Milk and Other Dairy Substitutes

If your kid likes cheesy, creamy, milky foods, there's a vegan variety for almost any cow-produced product. Many vegan cheeses have a way to go before they reach absolute equivalency in taste and melt-ability, but some—especially the vegan Parmesan and rice-based cheeses—have now moved far above the "just barely acceptable" culinary level. And milks like almond and many soy milks taste better and have a smoother texture than cow's milk.

❏ Almond milk

❏ Hazelnut milk

❏ Rice milk

❏ Soy milk (many flavors)

❏ Vegan cheese (many varieties)

❏ Vegan cream cheese

❏ Vegan Parmesan cheese

❏ Vegan sour cream

❏ Vegan whipped cream

❏ Vegan yogurt (soy- or coconut-based)

Parent Trap

Avoid quick-cooking rices, as they tend to be almost like white bread. Once kids get used to them, it's more difficult to get them to eat the heartier kinds.

Grains and Breads

Most kids won't like the more exotic grains such as quinoa, buckwheat groats, wild rice, and amaranth sometimes found in vegan recipes. Stick to the basics like rice and pasta, and introduce a few of the more kid-friendly grains listed here.

- ❏ Arborio rice
- ❏ Bagels
- ❏ Basmati rice
- ❏ Corn tortillas
- ❏ Couscous
- ❏ Flour tortillas
- ❏ Low-sugar breakfast cereals
- ❏ Oatmeal (quick and steel-cut)
- ❏ Old El Paso Spanish rice
- ❏ Orzo
- ❏ Pasta (semolina or whole-wheat)
- ❏ Pearled barley
- ❏ Pita bread
- ❏ Rice noodles
- ❏ Short-grain brown rice
- ❏ Tings
- ❏ Tortilla chips
- ❏ Vegan snack chips
- ❏ Whole-grain breads
- ❏ Whole-grain crackers

Beans

Some beans are worth buying canned, especially for busy parents who don't have time to soak and boil. Others, as noted here, are really worth the extra time due to improved quality, texture, and flavor.

Dried:

- ❏ Black beans
- ❏ Black-eyed peas
- ❏ Brown lentils
- ❏ Canary beans
- ❏ Green split peas
- ❏ Kidney beans
- ❏ Pinto beans
- ❏ Red lentils
- ❏ Small red beans
- ❏ Yellow lentils

Canned:

- ❏ Black beans
- ❏ Cannellini beans
- ❏ Garbanzo beans
- ❏ Pigeon peas
- ❏ Pinto beans
- ❏ Small red beans
- ❏ Vegetarian refried beans

Vegetables

The best way to encourage your kids to eat veggies is to serve them many ways. Some kids who like fresh, crisp veggies don't like them cooked and vice versa. Some will gobble up a salad with their favorite dressing, while others will only eat veggies in a soup, or frozen veggies. Keep trying!

- ❏ Baby carrots
- ❏ Baby salad greens
- ❏ Bell peppers
- ❏ Broccoli
- ❏ Cabbage (red and green)
- ❏ Cauliflower
- ❏ Celery
- ❏ Corn on the cob
- ❏ Cucumbers
- ❏ Frozen corn
- ❏ Frozen edamame
- ❏ Frozen peas
- ❏ Frozen pepper strips
- ❏ Frozen, prepared potatoes
- ❏ Garlic
- ❏ Iceberg lettuce
- ❏ Onions
- ❏ Potatoes (any variety)
- ❏ Snap peas
- ❏ Spinach
- ❏ String beans
- ❏ Vegan polenta

Fruits

Some kids are much more adventuresome than others when it comes to fruits. Here are some kid-approved standards. Avoid seedy fruits, as kids tend to dislike seeds, and younger children can choke on them. To quickly ripen hard fruits, place them in a paper bag with a banana.

Also, be sure to try the smaller, less starchy, baby banana as a new flavor twist on a daily standby fruit.

- ❏ Apples
- ❏ Applesauce (jarred)
- ❏ Apricots
- ❏ Avocadoes
- ❏ Bananas
- ❏ Blueberries

- ❑ Clementines
- ❑ Grapefruit
- ❑ Grapes (seedless)
- ❑ Kiwi
- ❑ Lemons
- ❑ Limes
- ❑ Local, seasonal fruits
- ❑ Mangoes
- ❑ Melons
- ❑ Oranges (seedless)

- ❑ Papayas
- ❑ Peaches (jarred, too)
- ❑ Pears (jarred, too)
- ❑ Pineapple
- ❑ *Plantains*
- ❑ Raspberries
- ❑ Strawberries
- ❑ Tangerines
- ❑ Watermelon

Vegan Vocab

Plantains, which resemble large bananas, are a fruit that can be fried, mashed, and cooked in many ways, especially when overripe. They're a good source of vitamins A and C as well as fiber.

Dried Fruits and Nuts

Dried fruits and nuts are healthy snacks. However, babies, toddlers, and kids with food allergies need to avoid most of these foods due to choking hazards or allergy risk.

Fruits:

- ❑ Dried apples
- ❑ Dried apricots
- ❑ Dried bananas
- ❑ Dried cranberries

- ❑ Dried mangoes
- ❑ Dried pineapple
- ❑ Raisins

Nuts:

❑ Almond butter

❑ Almonds

❑ Cashew butter

❑ Cashews

❑ Macadamia nuts

❑ Peanut butter

❑ Peanuts

❑ Pecans

❑ Pistachios

❑ Pumpkin seeds

❑ Sunflower seeds

❑ Tahini

❑ Walnuts

Other Canned and Dry Goods

Even if you have only a few basics in the fridge at the end of a week, keep these items stocked in your pantry, and you'll have everything you need to whip up a nearly gourmet meal—dessert included.

❑ Baking powder

❑ Baking soda

❑ Black (pitted) olives

❑ Blackstrap molasses

❑ Brown rice syrup

❑ Canned coconut milk

❑ Cranberry relish

❑ Diced tomatoes

❑ Dried onion soup mix

❑ Egg replacer

❑ Flour(s)

❑ Green (pitted) olives

❑ Jarred pizza sauce

❑ Jarred salsa (mild for most kids)

❑ Jarred vegan apple butter

❑ Nutritional yeast

❑ Oats

❑ Pickles

❑ Prepared vegan soups

❑ Stewed tomatoes

❑ Sugar(s)

❑ Tomato paste

❑ Tomato purée

❑ Tomato sauce

❑ Vegan chocolate chips

❑ Vegan mayo

❑ Veggie broth (low-sodium)

A word about flours and sugars: you can buy all-purpose, unbleached, whole-wheat, cake, garbanzo bean (great for a protein boost in baked goods), and rice flours, just to name a few. Usually, however, you'll want to use the kind specified in recipes, or the end result may not be the equivalent of the original intent.

If you or your child has gluten sensitivities, many excellent cookbooks are available that base their recipes on nonwheat flour. Start there, and experiment with substitutions in other standard wheat flour recipes when you get used to the textures and amounts in those specially formulated recipes.

We carefully placed the general word *sugar* on this pantry list knowing many types of sweeteners fall under the umbrella of this word: brown, white, confectioners', unbleached cane, agave, stevia, brown rice, Splenda, and more. Some vegans avoid using white and confectioners' sugar at all because much of it (but not all) is manufactured through a filtering process that uses animal bone char. We hope someday the refined white sugar that doesn't use the bone char process will be labeled "vegan" because some dessert recipes don't translate well with other forms of sweetener. Choose whatever form of sweetener you want for your baking, and substitute amounts according to package directions. But be aware that if your child is used to standard white refined sugar, the flavor of other sugars may be very noticeable to them until their taste buds adapt.

Oils, Vinegars, Spices, and Condiments

This isn't a comprehensive list by any means—but it is a kid-friendly one!

Oils and vinegars:

- ❏ Apple cider vinegar
- ❏ Asian sesame oil
- ❏ Balsamic vinegar
- ❏ Canola oil
- ❏ Crisco All-Vegetable Shortening
- ❏ Extra-virgin olive oil
- ❏ Nonstick spray oil
- ❏ Red wine vinegar
- ❏ Sunflower oil

Spices and condiments:

- ❏ Chutneys (mild varieties)
- ❏ Cinnamon
- ❏ Coriander
- ❏ Cumin
- ❏ Dijon mustard
- ❏ Dried basil
- ❏ Dried oregano

- ❏ Ginger
- ❏ Ketchup
- ❏ Kosher salt
- ❏ Mild curry powder
- ❏ Nutritional yeast
- ❏ Paprika
- ❏ Red cooking wine
- ❏ Salt substitutes
- ❏ Sea salt (use iodized salts)
- ❏ Soy sauce
- ❏ Vegan butter substitute
- ❏ Yellow mustard

> **Parent Trap**
>
> Salt substitutes, like the Mrs. Dash variety, can be an excellent way to introduce kids to spicy flavors without the use of salt.

Finding Food Allies

Vegan families now have a wide net of resources available. Natural food stores are among your best friends. Don't only frequent the national natural food chains; find your local natural food grocers as well. After a while, shopping at a local grocer often brings the added perks of them ordering special products you request or placing bulk orders for you. You may also benefit by attending cooking or health workshops held at local mom-and-pop shops. Sometimes the employees get to know your family and maybe even will drop a vegan treat in the bag at checkout for your child every now and again!

Ethnic grocers, such as Indian, Asian, Caribbean, and Latino, carry lots of specialty products often at lower prices than larger stores' ethnic sections because they sell more. Some ethnic grocers also sell prepared foods or know customers who make traditional foods—often vegan—you can buy and freeze to heat and eat.

Depending on where you live, nearby co-ops may carry locally grown organic produce, tofu, bulk grains, or shipments of nonperishable goods like canned foods that were rejected by mainstream grocers because of dented boxes or approaching expiration dates at extremely low cost.

Farmers' markets are the place to go to find fresh produce and connect with other families who care about their food choices and health. Kids especially enjoy seeing the farmers' wares and meeting the people who produce food near you. Some communities' farmers' markets may be more vegan-friendly than others. Check out yours and see.

> **That's So Vegan**
>
> You can have your very own "farmers' market" in your backyard by planting a small garden, even if it's just a few tomato plants, a window herb garden, or a strawberry patch. Kids love growing their own food!

Finally, tap in to the ever-growing number of online stores that cater to vegans (check out Appendix B for some addresses). It can be a bit more expensive because of shipping, but you can also find many foods, books, T-shirts, and other veg products you won't find elsewhere. Let your kids browse with you, and try a new product or two.

The Least You Need to Know

- Optimize the vegan grocery shopping experience by preplanning, making lists, organizing, and enlisting your family.

- To save money and please the crowd, don't get too fancy. Stick with kid-friendly pantry and fridge basics.

- Build a comprehensive grocery team from local grocery stores, health/natural food shops, ethnic grocers, farmers' markets, and online vegan specialty stores—and your own garden, too!

Chapter 11

Kids in the Kitchen

In This Chapter

- ◆ Kid-friendly kitchen tools
- ◆ Safety first
- ◆ Tips for little vegan chefs in training

The surest way to get your child excited about vegan food is to let her help you prepare it. Cooking is a time for her to sample fruits and veggies and watch as they change from raw to cooked, whole to juiced. She experiences firsthand what rice looks like uncooked, and how it transforms into the warm, fluffy stuff she loves. In effect, the kitchen becomes a yummy science lab!

From ages 2 to tween, kids can safely help make family meals, especially because all the uncooked meat and bacteria worries are out of the vegan kitchen. She can lick all the beaters in vegan recipes without the concern of salmonella in uncooked eggs!

In this chapter, we suggest some cool kitchen tools that will help make your kitchen easily adaptable to the special needs of little chefs. Of course, safe use of these tools and everything else in the kitchen is a must, so we've included a pre-food-prep checklist of safety musts to help keep your child from cutting or burning herself, slipping, falling, or anything else that would quickly turn a careless cooking moment from fun to fearful.

Next, choose from the age-appropriate lists of kid-friendly kitchen tasks to make your child enjoy cooking with you as much as you will appreciate her help! When you work together with your child preparing food—cleaning veggies and boiling beans with her rather than cracking eggs and broiling burgers—there's a lot of learning taking place through what she's doing, what you're talking about, and what's being prepared.

Tools of the Trade

No matter what her age, your child wants to play a part in the everyday workings of family life. Food preparation, serving, and cleanup is a huge part of daily family tasks.

Having the right *size* tools for the job is just as important as having the right tool for the job. With the right size tools, young children—even preschoolers—can begin to help clean and chop fruits and veggies (with parental supervision, of course). Kid-size zigzag vegetable slicers, banana slicers, vegetable brushes, self-enclosed onion choppers, and more make the work age-appropriate, fun, and safer than adult-size tools. One of our family favorites is a kid-size container with interchangeable lids for juicing, grating, and shredding.

That's So Vegan

You can find many kid-size kitchen and dining tools at online stores and catalogs that sell materials for families and schools that follow the Montessori Method, including the catalog at www.michaelolaf.com. Another great kid-friendly kitchen prop is The Learning Tower (www. mylearningtower.com), which helps kids ages 2 through 6 stand at adult countertop or table levels by raising them up safely on an adjustable, transportable wooden platform.

Other grown-up tools that are easy for kids to use (again, with parental supervision) include the following:

- Blenders (pressing the buttons)

- Cookie cutters and small butter spreaders (as a "knife" for cutting easily cut or spread foods like vegan margarine, bananas, vegan cream cheese, nut butters, dips, and spreads)

- Electric juicers (peeling and dropping in fruit)

- Garlic presses

- Measuring cups and spoons

- Nut choppers

- Pastry cutters

- Rolling pins

- Rubber scrapers

- Salad spinners

- Strainers (for cleaning off dried beans and legumes, and rinsing fruits and veggies)

- Vegetable peelers

Make cleanup part of the fun, too. Kids love to wear aprons, so be sure to make a special point of having your child's own apron hung near yours, and let her know the job's not done until the kitchen is clean and then the apron comes off! Buy a kid-size broom and mop. Add a bucket for hand-washing dishes at her level and another for filling up with compostables like peels for her to take out to the compost bin, and you have a clean kitchen!

Safety Features

The kitchen can be the most dangerous room in the house if you don't set up the cooking environment safely, and carefully assist your new chef in what she's doing if she's not old enough to cook on her own.

Experts say children under age 10 should not stay home alone, and that's probably a reasonable cut-off for allowing most children some level of freedom in the kitchen, too. Many kids may be able to microwave a premade vegan meal, make a piece of peanut butter and jelly toast, or even bake a batch of cookies on their own around age 10, but they may not be ready to operate the stovetop or a sharp knife with confidence until further into the teen years.

You know your child best and should be the judge when to extend these kitchen privileges by watching her master them many times with you present first. Go slowly, proceed with caution, check in, and be sure she knows all important safety rules before taking the next step up in the kitchen.

Here are some important cooking safety tips to go over with your child:

♦ Ask a parent's permission before making anything in the kitchen.

♦ Wash your hands, tie back your long hair, and pull up your sleeves before food preparation.

♦ Get on the correct height level for your workspace and what you're preparing. Being below counter height increases chances of spills.

♦ Don't plug in or turn on any kitchen appliance (juicer, blender, stove, toaster, mixer, etc.) without a parent's permission.

♦ Do not use the garbage disposal. Ever.

♦ Keep dishtowels, paper towels, and anything else that can catch fire away from the stove and other hot surfaces.

♦ Learn how to use a fire extinguisher (when age appropriate to cook alone).

♦ Follow recipe directions as precisely as possible.

Parent Trap

According to the U.S. Fire Administration, the most common reason for kitchen fires is leaving cooking food unattended. Check out more kitchen fire safety tips and a fun, short, kid's fire safety quiz at www.usfa.dhs.gov/kids.

◆ If you're not sure how to do something; if anything spills, breaks, oozes, or boils over; if you get cut, pinched, or burned; or if things just aren't going according to plan, ask your parent for help!

For you parents:

◆ Keep the handles on pans on the stove turned in so kids don't run into them, knock the pan off the stove, and get burned.

◆ Don't leave sharp knives resting on counters or sticking point up in the sink or dishwasher.

◆ Have an up-to-date fire extinguisher and fire alarm in the kitchen area.

◆ Wipe up spills right away to avoid slips or electrical issues.

◆ Keep household hot water heater between 120°F and 125°F to prevent scalding from the kitchen sink.

◆ Stay in the kitchen any time kids are using knives or appliances, or anytime the stove is on.

◆ Never let your child heat oil in a pan or make anything else that requires use of hot oil. If you're using hot oil or water on the stovetop, keep small children at least 3 feet away from the area.

These and other household safety rules should be reviewed each time you cook with your child. Consider printing these along with a list of your home's other kitchen rules to post on your refrigerator for constant reinforcement.

Jobs for Apprentice Chefs

When your child is just barely old enough to help you in the kitchen, the amount of time you spend *helping her* help you makes cooking time longer and more work. But those early years of training pay off well when she has a few more years of kitchen experience. The following sections outline some age-appropriate jobs you can expect your child to handle.

Ages 3 to 5

The littlest chefs in training can do a lot more in the kitchen than you might think—all with assistance, of course. Kids who help in the kitchen are not only helpful, having tons of fun, and learning skills like measuring and other math skills, but they're also much more likely to try new foods if they've helped prepare dinner.

Here are some pint-size jobs you could assign to your 3- to 5-year-old:

◆ Wash vegetables and fruits

◆ Slice a banana with a banana slicer

◆ Roll dough with a rolling pin

◆ Sprinkle vegan cheese on top of prepared sandwiches or tortillas

◆ Cut out cookies with cookie cutters

◆ Put fruit in a juicer or ingredients in a blender

◆ Mix batter with a spoon

◆ Wash beans and legumes in a strainer

◆ Chop nuts with an enclosed chopper

◆ Bring own dishes to the sink after meals

◆ Help wash dishes or empty dishwasher

◆ Unpack groceries from bags with the rest of the family

◆ Help sweep and mop floors

◆ Wipe off placemats

Ages 6 to 9

As a child gets older, especially if she's been your kitchen apprentice for a few years already, all those tasks listed for ages 3 to 5 will come naturally to her and she's ready to do them on her own. Stretch her kitchen know-how with the following new skills, helping as needed:

- Measure ingredients with cups and spoons

- Juice oranges with a manual juicer

- Slice veggies with a zigzag slicer

- Shred or grate with a child-size safety shredder/grater

- Peel easily peeled fruits and veggies with a safety peeler

- Cut and spread soft foods with a butter knife

- Mix batter with an electric mixer

- Set the table

- Microwave basic foods (with parental help)

- Pour drinks from small pitchers

- Put away groceries in appropriate cabinets or refrigerator bins

- Wipe down tables and countertops

Ages 10 to 12

Now's the time when all the prep work during the early years with your child in the kitchen pays off. In addition to all those tasks listed for ages 3 to 5 and 6 to 9, the following kitchen jobs will make your 10- to 12-year-old feel comfortable and confident enough in the kitchen to truly seem like your partner in cooking great vegan food—and even make herself simple meals on her own!

Standard safety rules apply, of course, and you need to know your child's unique cognitive developmental and emotional responsibility level before giving permission to make something on their own in the kitchen. Some of the jobs you may want to give them license to do at this age include:

- Read and execute basic recipes (no stovetop or sharp knives required), such as peanut butter cookies, with little or no help

- Flip pancakes and French toast (with supervision)

- De-seed vegetables like butternut squash

- Empty the dishwasher

- Mash potatoes

- Open cans with a handheld can opener

- Cut apples with a handheld corer/slicer

- Microwave basic foods

- Pour drinks from large pitchers

- Help younger kids make Play-Doh and other no-bake kitchen-based arts and crafts

- Within reason, make new food combinations for her own breakfast, lunch, or dinner (peanut butter, jelly, and potato chip sandwich, anyone?)

The Least You Need to Know

- From toddler to tween, kids can safely help make family meals in some small or large ways, especially because all the uncooked meat and bacteria worries are absent in the vegan kitchen.

- When kids are in the kitchen, supplying the right *size* tools for the job is just as important as having the right tools for the job.

- Set up the cooking environment safely, and carefully assist your child in what she's doing. Post a list of kitchen rules to reinforce safety.

- If you assign her age-appropriate tasks, you'll watch your child build confidence and a love of vegan cooking right before your eyes!

Part 4

Let's Eat!

Here comes the fun! In Part 4, we've included all the delicious vegan recipes the kids in our family—and even their nonvegan friends—have grown up loving. Find quick breakfast, lunch, snack, dinner, and dessert options, as well as a few more involved but definitely worth-the-time recipes.

It's our pleasure to share with you these recipes, as well as the tips and tricks we've learned from our own cooking trial and error, and from other vegan and vegetarian families and friends. From our kitchen to your table, enjoy!

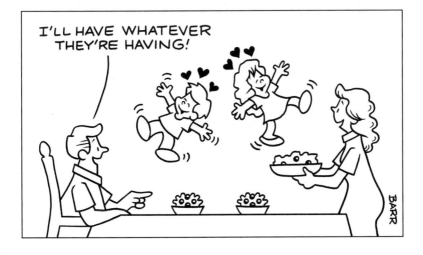

Chapter 12

Breakfasts They'll Wake Up For

In This Chapter

- ◆ The importance of breakfast
- ◆ Fast breakfasts to jump-start their day
- ◆ Slowing down for a vegan brunch

Breakfast is the most important meal of the day whether your child is vegan or not, because after about 12 hours without food, growing bodies need fuel. But before you start to worry about what you can serve your vegan child when the "usual" eggs, bacon, and pancakes are out of the picture, relax. In this chapter, we give you ideas and recipes for lots of vegan kid-friendly breakfast favorites.

It's estimated that as many as 48 percent of American girls and 32 percent of boys don't eat breakfast every day. For most families, it simply comes down to having no time to sit and eat before rushing out the door to before school practices and early morning meetings. In the following pages, we share some ideas for nutritious breakfasts on the run. And for mornings when you have more time, check out our delicious family brunch suggestions. And don't forget breakfast for dinner every once in a while can make for easy evening meals and fun family memories.

The Most Important Meal of the Day

Wake up and smell the coffee! Breakfast is crucial to a healthful life-style for all kids and adults. Skipping breakfast has been strongly linked to the development of obesity, and studies show that overweight and obese children, adolescents, and adults are less likely to eat breakfast than their thinner counterparts.

Kids who don't eat a healthful breakfast each morning tend to pull lower test scores, and understandably so. It's hard to concentrate when you're hungry, and kids who don't eat breakfast will be hungry. Some breakfast skippers also have behavioral problems in school. Many kids who start the day with nutrient deficits never make up for them in later meals of the day.

Even if your child does eat breakfast, it must be healthful to be effective. If the food he eats first thing in the morning is full of sugar and low on protein and complex carbs, like doughnuts, his blood sugar will take a nasty swing, his mood will likely swing right along with it, and he'll be hungry again within hours. So prepare in advance. Plan breakfast the night before. Choose a few breakfast options at the grocery store that you can make the night before, pack in a paper bag, and eat in the car on those really harried mornings.

If your child doesn't like to eat breakfast, he still needs to do so. Wake him up earlier, and encourage a shower and maybe a walk with the dog to help wake up his body before breakfast. Maybe he just dislikes breakfast foods, so offer a more traditionally lunch or dinner food at breakfast. If all else fails, toss a vegan snack bar at your child as he leaves

Parent Trap

Don't rely on the school breakfast option to give your child a healthful morning meal on a regular basis. Even if it may be better than no breakfast at all, many of the at-school breakfast programs pack a sugar punch, with cinnamon rolls and other sugary breakfast "treats."

for school. He can nibble on it as he enters school or between classes. Younger kids typically have a snack time in the morning at school, so pack a big, calorie- and nutrient-dense one if he doesn't currently chow down at home in the morning.

Quick Starts

As parents ourselves, we hear you. You want (some might say *need!*) some speedy breakfasts for those mornings when your child is barely out of his pajamas 15 minutes before the school bell rings. We've got you covered.

Smoothies are the fastest, healthiest way to start the day quickly! If you have a blender, homemade fruit smoothies are as vegan, homemade, natural, healthful, and transportable as you can get in less than 5 minutes. Adding extras like flaxseed oil, protein powder, silken tofu, vegan yogurt, or peanut or other nut butters can boost the nutrient benefits even further. Check out *The Ultimate Smoothie Book* by Cherie Calbom for many vegan and vegan-adaptable smoothie recipes. Buy a few premade, all-natural smoothies (check to be sure they're dairy-free) at your local natural foods store to have on hand in case of a really rushed day.

Fruit won't be enough on its own to keep most kids fueled for an entire morning. But in a pinch, a banana paired with a handful of nuts, or an apple, some grapes, or a peach paired with a slice of pumpkin bread gives a good start to the day.

Cereal can often be surprisingly vegan (although it's unlikely that the vitamin-fortified nutrients in the cereal are all vegan-sourced, but go for the BPO here). Go for the whole-grain, low-sugar varieties. Our favorite milk with cereal is rice milk because it's light and seems to make cereal stay crispy longer than the heavier soy or nut versions. But experiment with your child's favorites. If he will eat cereal with calcium-fortified soy milk, just 1 cup can provide most of his daily calcium needs and some B_{12} as well.

A nut-butter-and-jelly sandwich is an all-time kid favorite. Experiment with different nut butters beyond peanut. Expand your child's jelly and jam selections from grape and strawberry with new flavors like raspberry, blueberry, peach, rhubarb, and apricot. (To be sure it's vegan, look for pectin, not gelatin.) Or thinly slice a banana into the sandwich. If storing in a quick-take bag overnight, lay a piece of waxed paper between the jelly/jam and the bread to prevent mushy bread.

Parent Trap

Beware the bread. Many manufactured breads contain milk or milk derivatives and honey. Very few mass-marketed breads exclude these nonvegan ingredients, but your local natural foods store might have some options for you. Or you could make your own!

Cold pancake sandwiches can serve as an inventive twist to Monday morning breakfast if you have some leftover vegan pancake batter from Sunday brunch. Make up the rest of the batter after brunch, and store the pancakes in the fridge. In the morning, slather some nut butter and a tiny drizzle of syrup on top, fold in half, and go.

Leftovers can work for breakfast, too. If last night's meal was one of your child's favorites, don't be shy about warming it up and serving it this morning. There's no rule that says dinner can't be breakfast every now and again.

Bagel sandwiches are relatively easy and a quick warm breakfast. Toast two halves of a bagel, spread thinly with vegan cream cheese, add a microwaved soy sausage cut in half lengthwise, drizzle with maple syrup, and you've got a simple and delicious breakfast.

Soy or coconut yogurt are transportable—just don't forget the spoon! Some soy-based yogurts do contain dairy, so check the label. Coconut milk–based yogurt comes in individual serving size cartons and can be absolutely delicious.

Muffins and quick breads can be sugary, fatty morning downers, or good sources of fiber, iron, and protein, depending on the ingredients. Check labels, or again, make your own.

Energy-style bars can become pricey if you rely on them too much for quick meals and snacks, but they do work to quickly quell hunger and meet nutritional needs. Stock some vegan bars in your pantry and in the car, in case you run out of the house and remember breakfast halfway to school!

Almost all these quick breakfast ideas can be stored in the fridge the night before, paired with a juice box or bottle of water, and put in a sack with a handful of nuts and a multivitamin for a portable breakfast your child can eat on the bus or in the car on the way to school.

That's So Vegan _____

No scientific evidence shows one time of day is better than another for taking a multivitamin most effectively. But if you give your child his multivitamin first thing in the morning, you're most likely to remember. Another consideration: iron is more readily absorbed when eaten with vitamin C–rich foods.

Vegan Brunches

The time to get fancy with vegan breakfast foods is at brunch. Brunches are fabulous family breakfast-lunch combos after a sleepover, on a relaxed weekend day, or for a special holiday that suits itself to a special meal early in the day.

Brunch can be as easy as a pancake/waffle bar—complete with sliced bananas, strawberries, and blueberries; chopped nuts; chocolate chips; three kinds of syrup; and vegan whipped cream. Or it can get as elaborate (yet remain kid-friendly) as a first course of a mixed fresh fruit salad with vegan muffins; a second course of scrambled tofu, veggie bacon, and roasted red potatoes; and brunch "dessert" of vegan cream cheese and fruit–stuffed French toast cut into finger sandwiches. Freshly squeezed juice gains any brunch at least two stars.

For more brunch ideas, check out *Vegan Brunch: Homestyle Recipes Worth Waking Up For—From Asparagus Omelets to Pumpkin Pancakes* by Isa Chandra Moskowitz.

Sweetened Steel-Cut Oats

This warm, nutty, almost brown rice–esque oatmeal takes on the sweet flavor of maple syrup and soy milk, making the heartiness of this powerhouse food more palatable to kids.

1 cup water

¼ cup *steel-cut oats*

1 cup plain soy milk

2 TB. pure maple syrup

2 TB. walnuts or pecans

2 TB. raisins, chopped dried apricots, dried apples, or dates

Yield: 2 servings
Prep time:
5 minutes
Cook time:
20 to 25 minutes
Serving size:
1 cup

1. In a small saucepan over high heat, bring water to a boil. Pour in oatmeal and stir.

2. When oatmeal begins to thicken, reduce heat to low, cover, and simmer for 15 to 20 minutes, removing lid to stir occasionally.

3. Remove from heat, and divide oatmeal into 2 bowls. Over each bowl, pour ½ cup soy milk, drizzle 1 tablespoon maple syrup, and sprinkle 1 tablespoon walnuts or pecans and 1 tablespoon preferred dried fruit. Serve immediately.

Vegan Vocab

Steel-cut oats are the least processed of any form of oatmeal. Many people find the taste and texture of these oats far superior to other forms of oatmeal, but if your child is new to oatmeal or not a huge fan, you may want to start with the quick oats and gradually move to the heartier version of oats. Once you get hooked on steel-cut oats, regular oatmeal tastes and feels far too wimpy!

Kids' Scrambled Tofu

The hearty texture of extra-firm tofu mixed with zesty yellow curry and soy sauce and topped with a sprinkle of melted vegan cheese is simple enough to please even the pickiest kids.

1 (2-lb.) pkg. extra-firm tofu

1 tsp. sea salt

2 tsp. turmeric

1 tsp. mild yellow curry powder

2 TB. low-sodium soy sauce or Bragg's Liquid Amino Acids

2 TB. olive oil

$\frac{1}{4}$ cup vegan rice-based cheese

Yield: 4 to 6 servings
Prep time: 10 minutes
Cook time: 10 minutes
Serving size: About 1 cup

1. Drain and dry block of tofu by wrapping it in paper towels and squeezing over the sink. Using your hands, crumble tofu into a medium bowl.

2. Add sea salt, turmeric, yellow curry, and soy sauce, and stir gently until blended.

3. In a high-sided cast-iron skillet over medium-high heat, add olive oil. Add tofu mixture and sauté for 5 to 10 minutes or until some of the tofu has browned nicely. (Don't sauté until too much tofu gets browned, however; you want more egglike chewy tofu than browned.)

4. Sprinkle top of tofu with rice cheese (if using), reduce heat to low, cover, and allow cheese to melt.

5. Serve immediately.

That's So Vegan

Many scrambled tofu recipes include vegetables such as mushrooms, bell peppers, diced onions, and chunks of sautéed zucchini kids turn up their noses at. Ours leaves those out. For the veggie-loving adults, sauté these veggies (or your favorites) in a separate pan and mix them in after the plain portions have been dished out, topped with diced fresh tomato and a leaf or two of fresh basil.

Tortilla Wraps

Leftover Kids' Scrambled Tofu creates a chewy center for these crispy breakfast tortillas served with mild salsa and vegan sour cream.

1 (8-in.) flour tortilla

$\frac{1}{2}$ cup Kids' Scrambled Tofu (recipe earlier in this chapter)

$\frac{1}{4}$ cup grated vegan rice cheddar cheese

1 TB. mild salsa

1 TB. vegan sour cream

Yield: 1 serving
Prep time: 5 minutes
Cook time: 4 to 6 minutes
Serving size: 1 wrap

1. Spray a cast-iron skillet with nonstick cooking spray, and lay flour tortilla in the skillet.

2. In a medium bowl, mix tofu and rice cheese with a spoon. Spread tofu mixture onto center of tortilla.

3. Fold $\frac{1}{3}$ tortilla onto itself to center, and place 3 or 4 shreds of rice cheese on edge of tortilla to create a seal as you fold the other $\frac{1}{3}$ on that side. Turn tortilla seam side down.

4. Cook over medium heat for 2 or 3 minutes. Gently flip over tortilla, and cook 2 or 3 more minutes. Remove tortilla from skillet, and serve with salsa and vegan sour cream.

That's So Vegan

If your child doesn't like salsa, try substituting something sweet such as diced fresh peaches or mango or a mild, jarred salsa. Or try the Newman's Own brand salsas that contain peaches or pineapple.

Puffy Pancakes

These yummy pancakes are incredibly fluffy and light. Add blueberries or chocolate chips for extra-cool parent points!

1 cup unbleached all-purpose flour

1 TB. sugar or equivalent sugar alternative

1 TB. plus 1 tsp. baking powder

$\frac{1}{2}$ tsp. salt

Egg replacer equivalent to 2 eggs, prepared according to pkg. directions

1 cup rice milk

2 TB. sunflower or other light vegetable oil

Yield: 8 to 10 small pancakes, 4 or 5 servings

Prep time:
10 minutes

Cook time:
1 or 2 minutes per batch

Serving size:
2 pancakes

1. In a large bowl, combine flour, sugar, baking powder, and salt.

2. In a medium bowl, combine prepared egg replacer, rice milk, and sunflower oil.

3. Add liquid mixture to dry ingredients, and stir, leaving some lumpiness. Let sit for at least 5 minutes, or longer if you have more time.

4. Coat a cast-iron skillet with 1 tablespoon vegan margarine, and set over medium-high heat. Pour about 2 tablespoons batter into heated skillet for each pancake. Turn pancakes over when bubbles on top begin to break.

5. When bottom of pancake firms (test with a spatula) but is not too dark or crisp, remove from pan. Serve immediately with syrup, sliced fresh fruit, and even a few vegan chocolate chips.

That's So Vegan

The key to making light and fluffy vegan pancakes is to let the batter sit for as long as possible to give the baking powder time to work its magic. It also helps to make the pancakes silver dollar size. Larger pancakes tend to be more dense and hard to cook evenly through.

Punkin'-Raisin Bread

Moist, sweet, and cinnamon-spicy, this bread sprinkled with plump, juicy raisins will soon become a family favorite.

Egg replacer equal to 2 eggs, prepared according to pkg. directions

$\frac{1}{3}$ cup canola or other light vegetable oil

$\frac{1}{3}$ cup rice milk

1 cup canned pumpkin

2 cups unbleached all-purpose flour

1 cup firmly packed light brown sugar

2 TB. baking powder

1 tsp. baking soda

$\frac{1}{2}$ tsp. pumpkin pie spice

$\frac{1}{4}$ tsp. salt

2 tsp. cinnamon

$\frac{1}{2}$ cup raisins

2 TB. walnuts (optional)

Yield: 1 loaf
Prep time:
30 minutes
Cook time:
40 minutes
Serving size:
1 (2-inch) slice

1. Preheat the oven to 400°F. Spray the bottom of a 9×5-inch metal bread loaf pan with cooking spray.

2. In a large bowl, combine egg replacer, oil, rice milk, and pumpkin. Add 1 cup flour, brown sugar, baking powder, baking soda, pumpkin pie spice, salt, and cinnamon. With an electric mixer on medium speed, beat for 2 minutes or until well blended.

3. Add remaining 1 cup flour and raisins, and mix with a wooden spoon. Pour batter into the prepared pan, keeping the sides of the pan as clean of batter drips as possible.

4. Bake for 40 minutes. Test doneness by inserting a knife into bread. If it comes out clean, it's done.

5. Remove from oven. Poke walnuts into the top of loaf (if using, keep one side walnut-free for kids who don't like walnuts). Let sit for about 5 minutes, remove from pan, and cool completely on a wire rack.

That's So Vegan

For a perfect car-ready, on-the-way-to school breakfast, wrap up a slice of Punkin'-Raisin Bread, add in a single-serve cup of soy or coconut yogurt, and fill a water bottle with some juice. That's a healthier, yummier breakfast than any drive-thru could ever dream to have.

Fruit Soup

The flavors in this light and easy but nutritious breakfast soup are reminiscent of fresh summer berries and cream desserts.

1 peach, nectarine, pear, banana (peeled), or other soft fruit, sliced

½ cup fresh berries

1 cup soy milk, rice milk, or almond milk

1 tsp. brown sugar

Yield: 1 serving
Prep time:
5 minutes
Serving size:
2 or 3 cups

1. Place sliced fruit and berries in a cereal bowl, and cover with milk.

2. Sprinkle with brown sugar, and serve.

Parent Trap

Especially when using unpeeled fruits, be sure they're organic. Check out Chapter 10 for a list of must-buy organic fruits and veggies.

Berry Breakfast Smoothie

This smoothie is rich, thick, and sweet. The sweetness of the berries and soy (or nut) milk will make your child forget all about the healthful stuff in there like flax and protein powder!

1 cup almond or vanilla soy milk

3 to 5 medium ice cubes

2 TB. vegan protein powder (preferably soy-free)

1 TB. flaxseed powder

$\frac{1}{4}$ cup frozen blueberries

Yield: 1 smoothie
Prep time:
3 minutes
Serving size:
$1\frac{1}{2}$ cups

1. In a blender, add almond milk and ice cubes. Add protein powder, flaxseed powder, and frozen blueberries.

2. Blend on high speed (or auto ice crusher mode, if you have one on your blender), for 2 minutes or until smooth.

3. Pour into a to-go cup, stick in a wide straw, and go!

That's So Vegan

This smoothie contains protein powder to keep kids' bellies filled for the long morning at school. Substitute any of your child's favorite blendable fruit for the frozen blueberries, and use organic whenever possible. Some kids notice the flaxseed powder more than others. If your child really doesn't like it, you can easily omit it.

Chapter 13

Lunches to Love

In This Chapter

- ◆ Super school lunches
- ◆ Perfect play date lunches, whether you host or not
- ◆ Easy lunches on the run

For school-age kids, lunchtime often means eating away from home. Whether your child is at school, at a friends' house, on the road, or just outside enjoying the noonday sun, her vegan lunches need to be portable, quick to eat, and nonperishable. Younger kids still at home have more lunchtime options. For these little ones, the goal is to serve food at lunch you can adapt for your own midday meal and that's low in sugar and filling so naptime comes easily. If your solid-food eating child is in daycare, you'll likely want to pack a vegan lunch for her, as most child-care providers probably won't fully accommodate vegan lunches unless you provide them (see Chapter 3 for child care–specific advice).

In this chapter, we help you "do lunch" for your little ones, thanks to our easy and do-able lunch ideas and recipes.

The Envy of the Lunchroom

More than likely, your vegan child will need to bring lunch to school, at least when no veg option is offered (or when she's tired of the daily salad bar). These days, there's no reason school lunches need to be cold or bagged. With an amazing array of fun lunchboxes and thermoses (check out www.laptoplunches.com for some of our favorites), you can pack warm lunches you can rest assured will stay warm until your little one's ready to eat.

At the beginning of the school year, we brainstorm ideas for what they would like to try in their lunchboxes. Along with our own ideas, we print out the list at www. vegcooking.com/backtoschool.asp, and the kids check off the choices that sound appealing. Some ideas are hits; others don't get a passing grade after our kids try them. But we have come up with a core group of about 10 healthful, packable lunches that can be easily rotated throughout the year with an occasional hot lunch.

Vegan Voices

Keep it simple. I don't send my son off to school with a lunchbox of falafel or chana masala if he doesn't want it. Pizza! Fruit! Chips! Carrots! Fun!

—Michael, Virginia

Here are some of our kids' favorite school lunch ideas:

◆ Veggies with hummus dip

◆ Cold pasta salads

◆ A-B-Vegan Soup (recipe later in this chapter) with garlic bagel

◆ Baby carrots, garbanzo beans, and spiced almonds

◆ Vegetarian baked beans with veggie dogs cut up and mixed in a thermos

◆ Leftover barbecue tofu strips

◆ Any of Amy's Kitchen brand vegan soups

Don't stick to the mundane apple or banana in the lunchbox every day! An amazingly diverse assortment of packaged fruits and veggies are available in mainstream grocery stores these days. From packaged pineapple spears to dried peas and carrots, your child need never get bored with a plant-based lunch.

Play Date Lunches

It's simple to serve omnivorous kids vegan food without fuss when you're the play date host. In our experience, most of our children's non-veg friends love the chance to try veggie chicken nuggets or baked tofu cubes and sides of fresh fruit, fun-shaped pasta with vegan margarine, and vegan cookies for dessert. It's a novelty to them, and most kids love trying new and different ways of doing things, if only to go home and shock their parents with the news that they ate tofu and lived to tell the tale! Or if you want to serve something "tamer" you can always go with vegan tacos, vegan mac and cheese, and pita pizzas.

When your child leaves the nest for her first play dates out, unless the host family is also vegan, it's a good idea to pack your child a lunch (with a vegan treat to share with her friend). Having taken this preemptive step, there's no hot seat for your child left to climb off alone when the cheeseburger or turkey sandwich is served and you're not present.

As your child gets older, leave it up to her whether she wants to take food when she goes over to hang out at friends' houses. She may prefer it, or especially in the tween years it may be embarrassing or isolating. Perhaps she'd rather just eat the few veg-appropriate foods served at the friend's house, like fruit or chips, and eat more upon returning home. Respect her comfort level and social needs.

Out to Lunch

School isn't the only place kids find themselves out and about at lunch-time. Eating while out and about or especially when traveling can sometimes present challenges for vegans of all ages.

Vegan bars, dried fruit, and nuts lend themselves well to days out. Don't forget the bottled water! Infants and young children become dehydrated much more quickly than teens and adults. If your child is active in sports, encourage hydration by bringing water bottles with you. Or provide water-rich fruits and veggies as snacks at half-time and afterward for hydration.

That's So Vegan

Check out www. happycow.net for a global (yes, *global*) guide to veg-friendly restaurants and health food stores. Add your favorites, too!

When traveling, it might be easiest to pack your own veg foods. (Taco Bell's bean burritos minus the cheese is one of the few vegan fast-food options other than salads.) If you're flying, be careful about packing travel snacks. Liquid snacks like smoothies, juice boxes, or sippy cups filled with liquid of any kind won't make it through security.

Travel is one of those times that settling for the BPO may be necessary. Still, you can try to avoid BPO situations by packing more food for your child than you think necessary. Especially on long road trips, pack the biggest cooler you can fit in your car. You'll not only have food for the road, you'll also have room to pack food to eat when you get to the nonvegan relative's house, hotel, or wherever you happen to be going.

Christi's Secret-Ingredient Hummus

This hummus is kid-friendly because the onions and garlic are sautéed, leaving a much milder taste that comes from the secret ingredient— tahini-based jarred salad dressing.

2 tsp. olive oil

1 small sweet onion, finely diced

3 to 5 cloves garlic, minced

$\frac{1}{2}$ cup tahini

$\frac{1}{2}$ cup Annie's Goddess Dressing, or other tahini-based salad dressing

$\frac{1}{2}$ cup lemon juice

1 tsp. cumin

1 tsp. salt

3 cups canned garbanzo beans, drained and rinsed

Yield: 4 cups
Prep time: 30 minutes
Cook time: 5 minutes
Serving size: $\frac{1}{4}$ to $\frac{1}{2}$ cup

1. In a small saucepan or skillet over medium-high heat, heat olive oil. Add onion, and cook for 2 or 3 minutes. Add garlic, and cook for 1 more minute or until onions are soft. (Reduce the heat if garlic begins to brown, which you don't want.)

2. In a deep medium bowl, mix tahini, Annie's Goddess Dressing, lemon juice, cumin, and salt. Add cooked onions and garlic.

3. Pour in garbanzo beans. Mash with a potato masher until desired consistency.

4. Serve fresh at room temperature, or chill and serve with crackers, veggies, on sandwiches, or alongside cold pasta or bagels.

That's So Vegan

Get the kiddos involved by juicing the lemons or dicing the onions with a blade-enclosed hand food chopper. To give some earthy chunkiness to the hummus—which makes it heartier on bagels or in pitas and other sandwiches—leave some halves and quarters of garbanzo beans unmashed. For creamy, smooth hummus, pour all the ingredients into a blender or food processor and blend until smooth.

Tofu Dunkers

These crunchy little baked tofu bites are delicious dunked in tahini, mustard, barbecue sauce, or soy sauce.

1 (1-lb.) pkg. extra- or super-firm tofu

Olive oil–based nonstick cooking spray

$\frac{1}{2}$ tsp. coarse kosher salt

Yield: 5 servings
Prep time:
10 minutes
Cook time:
20 minutes
Serving size:
7 nuggets

1. Preheat the oven to 400°F. Spray a 12×18-inch baking sheet with cooking spray.

2. Drain and dry block of tofu by wrapping it in paper towels and squeezing over the sink. Cut tofu into 1-inch cubes. Arrange in a single layer on the prepared baking sheet.

3. Lightly spray tops of tofu cubes with cooking spray, and sprinkle salt evenly over all.

4. Bake for 10 minutes, flip tofu with a spatula, and cook for 10 more minutes.

5. Remove tofu from the baking sheet onto a paper towel–lined plate, cover with another paper towel, and blot to remove excess salt and oil.

6. Wait 5 to 10 minutes for interior of tofu to cool before serving.

That's So Vegan

These baked tofu cubes are a great addition to many dishes, including curries, stir-fries, pasta, and casseroles, and they're much lower in fat than pan- or deep-fried tofu. For tofu sandwiches, simply slice the uncooked tofu block into fourths lengthwise and prepare and bake the same way as the cubes.

A-B-Vegan Soup

This hearty yet mildly flavored tomato-veggie-pasta soup will be a hit with kids of all ages, even toddlers.

2 TB. olive oil

1 small yellow onion, very finely chopped

2 cloves garlic, minced

8 cups vegetable broth

1 (28-oz.) can stewed tomatoes, with juice

3 small-medium white potatoes, peeled and cubed

1 medium carrot, peeled and diced

1 cup shredded green cabbage

1 tsp. chopped fresh basil

1 cup alphabet pasta

1 cup frozen yellow corn

1 or 2 cups canned cannellini beans, rinsed and drained

Yield: 8 servings
Prep time:
15 minutes
Cook time:
About 50 minutes
Serving size:
2 cups

1. In a 5-quart saucepan over medium heat, heat olive oil. Add onion and garlic, and sauté for about 2 to 4 minutes or until onions are translucent but garlic isn't burned.

2. Pour in vegetable broth, and add stewed tomatoes (break apart large lumps with a spoon), potatoes, carrot, cabbage, and basil. Bring to a boil, reduce heat to medium-low, cover, and cook for 30 minutes.

3. Meanwhile, cook pasta in a separate pan according to package directions. Drain when finished.

4. Add cooked pasta, corn, and beans to soup. Let corn and beans warm for 5 to 10 minutes, and serve.

That's So Vegan

There's something about little pasta letters that changes a soup from a boring vegetable soup to a fun lunchtime spelling activity!

Vegan Pasta Salad

The bright colors and sweet, zesty flavors absolutely burst out of this beautiful pasta salad that's a winner at picnics and potlucks or in your child's lunch box.

1 (16-oz.) box bow tie, campanelle, shells, rotini, or radiatori pasta

1 TB. olive oil

1 large red bell pepper, ribs and seeds removed, and cut into long, thin slices

1 or 2 large garlic cloves, minced

2 cups fresh spinach, torn into small pieces

1 cup frozen petite lima beans

$\frac{1}{2}$ cup black olives

4 jarred artichoke hearts, quartered

2 TB. extra-virgin olive oil

2 TB. red wine vinegar

1 TB. white granulated sugar or sugar substitute equivalent

1 large or 2 or 3 small carrots, peeled and shredded

$\frac{1}{2}$ cup vegan Parmesan cheese

Yield: 10 cups
Prep time:
About 30 minutes
Cook time:
35-40 minutes
Serving size:
$\frac{1}{2}$ to 1 cup

1. Prepare pasta according to the package directions, and drain. Set aside in very large bowl to cool.

2. Meanwhile, in a cast-iron skillet over medium-high heat, heat 1 tablespoon olive oil. Add red bell pepper, and sauté for 2 minutes or until pepper is soft. Add garlic and spinach, reduce heat to medium, and sauté for 1 minute or so more until garlic is cooked and spinach is wilted but garlic is not browned.

3. Add frozen lima beans, sautéed veggies, olives, and artichokes to pasta.

4. In small bowl, mix extra-virgin olive oil, red wine vinegar, and sugar. Pour dressing over pasta-veggie mix, and stir to coat all ingredients with dressing.

5. In a pinch, serve as is, or refrigerate for at least 30 minutes or until cool. Just before serving, top with shredded carrots and vegan Parmesan cheese.

> **That's So Vegan**
>
> If your child dislikes any of the veggies in this pasta salad, cut them in larger pieces so they can easily be removed, or set them in nearby ramekins for adults and other kids to add in. Otherwise, pack in all you can!

Veggie Chix Salad Sandwich

Mild curry brings an ethnic flavor to this typically American fare, and the apple offers a sweet surprise.

1 (8-oz.) pkg. meat analog chicken strips

6 TB. vegan mayo

2 tsp. mild yellow curry powder

1 TB. orange juice

½ cup red or green apple, diced, peel on

4 to 6 whole-wheat pita pockets (half-moon shape)

> **Yield: 4 to 6 sandwiches**
>
> **Prep time:**
> 25 minutes
>
> **Cook time:**
> 5 minutes
>
> **Serving size:**
> 1 filled pita pocket

1. Cook chicken strips according to package directions. Remove from heat, and let cool.

2. Meanwhile, in small bowl, blend mayo and curry with a spoon. Add orange juice, and fold in chicken strips and apple. Refrigerate for 10 minutes before stuffing pita pockets.

> **That's So Vegan**
>
> If you like, you can substitute extra-firm tofu for the chicken strips in this recipe. Simply coarsely crumble it, and mix it in.

3. Evenly divide apple mixture among pita pockets, and serve.

Pita Pizzas

These fast, warm, and filling pita pizzas feature a crispy pita crust; cheesy, saucy topping; and your favorite extra toppings.

4 half-moon whole-wheat pita pockets

4 TB. jarred vegan pizza sauce

$\frac{1}{2}$ to $\frac{3}{4}$ cup shredded rice mozzarella cheese

Your choice pizza toppings (black or green olives, canned or fresh mushrooms, veggie pepperoni, thinly sliced vegan Italian sausage, thinly sliced green bell pepper, or onion)

Yield: 4 pita pizzas
Prep time:
4 minutes
Cook time:
14 minutes
Serving size:
1 pita pizza

1. Preheat the oven to 350°F. Line a baking sheet with aluminum foil.

2. Arrange pita pockets in a single layer on the foil, and spread 1 tablespoon sauce on each. Evenly sprinkle vegan cheese on each, and add any desired toppings.

3. Bake for 10 to 13 minutes. If necessary, transfer cooked pitas to a microwave-safe plate and microwave for 1 minute to completely melt cheese.

That's So Vegan

The crusts for these speedy pizzas are whole-wheat pitas, which provide 4 grams protein, 4 grams fiber, and only 1 gram fat. Try to buy pita pockets enriched with flax for a good source of omega-3s, too. Freeze leftover pitas for up to 3 months, keep an extra jar of vegan pizza sauce in the pantry and some vegan mozzarella cheese in the fridge, and you have an instant last-minute play date meal kids can help prepare.

How-Many-Layers? Burritos

Tropical flavors and hearty textures stuff these burritos as full as you and your child choose to make them.

2 cups cooked basmati, brown, or boxed vegan Spanish rice

4 (8-in.) flour tortillas

$^1/_2$ cup vegan refried beans

1 cup vegan shredded cheddar cheese

Your choice layers (avocados, pitted and sliced black or green olives, tomatoes, mangoes, pickled jalapeño peppers or carrots, or canned mild green chiles)

$^1/_2$ cup vegan sour cream

1 cup iceberg lettuce, shredded

Yield: 4 burritos
Prep time:
10 to 20 minutes
Cook time:
25 minutes
Serving size:
1 burrito

1. Cook rice according to package directions. Drain if necessary.

2. Spread $^1/_2$ of one side of each tortilla with 1 tablespoon refried beans, $^1/_4$ cup vegan cheddar cheese, $^1/_2$ cup rice, and any other toppings you like. Wrap $^1/_3$ of tortilla onto itself, and sprinkle with a few shreds of cheese to seal as you wrap the other $^1/_3$ on top of that.

3. Spray a cast-iron skillet with high-heat nonstick vegetable spray, and heat over medium-high heat. Add burritos to the pan, and fry for 3 minutes. Flip over burritos, and fry for 2 more minutes.

4. Remove burritos from the pan, and place on individual plates. Open slowly to allow steam to escape. (Burritos will be hot!) Spread 1 tablespoon vegan sour cream on inside flap of each tortilla, sprinkle $^1/_4$ cup lettuce in each center, and allow each person to layer individual burrito with cold fillings (avocados, tomatoes, mangoes, for example). Serve with salsa and more vegan sour cream if desired.

That's So Vegan

Have a competition with your kids and count who has the highest number of layers in their burrito (nine is our family's record-size burrito). Now *that's* what we call healthy competition!

Chapter 14

Delicious Dinners

In This Chapter

- ◆ Sit-down vegan dinners
- ◆ Vegan for the holidays
- ◆ Parties, potlucks, and cookouts, vegan-style

Mealtime is a great time to reconnect and refuel—as long as everyone's happily eating! If you have unhappy eaters at the dinner table, power struggles are bound to happen. Our wish for your family is that the words "You will sit here until you eat all that tofu loaf!" will never be uttered at dinnertime in your home again. The trick is to find vegan meals that are simple to make, that are healthful, and that everyone likes.

This chapter supplies ideas for easy dinners at home, including quick weeknight buffet-style dinners, one-pot dinners, down-home comfort foods, and our family's holiday favorites. We also suggest some crowd-pleasing appetizers, potluck favorites, and tips on navigating the next neighborhood cookout.

So ring the bell, have a seat, and grab your fork. It's dinnertime!

Peaceful Family Meal Times

According to recent studies, kids whose families eat meals together more often than not have better physical and mental health, perform at a higher level in school, and are happier teens than kids whose families don't eat together often. Also, it may be common sense simply proven by studies, but we now know that kids pick up most of their attitudes about eating from their parents. The kinds of foods you eat, your portion sizes, and your attitudes about eating impact your child's choices more than anyone else's. Vegan parents, that's good news!

That said, most kids have their own distinct taste and texture preferences and may not always like what's for dinner. Be flexible. The best vegan family recipes are ones that include ingredients that kids can easily leave off or take out of their plate or bowl, or that the adults can add in after cooking a milder version for the kiddos. For example, a dinnertime taco or burrito bar is a great way to give your picky eater the option of just beans, rice, and vegan cheese in her taco, while giving the more adventuresome kids and adults free reign to stuff jalapeños, lettuce, tomatoes, olives, caramelized onions, and taco sauce in with the beans and rice.

If dinner consists of a recipe your child dislikes, serve some of his favorite side dishes that nutritionally equal the main dish. Say you're serving lentil loaf, which everyone in your family but him likes. You know he loves mashed potatoes and steamed broccoli, so make them the evening's side dishes. Add a veggie tray and some whole-wheat crackers with his favorite cashew butter or hummus dip, serve a fruit-based dessert, and you've got a balanced meal with no arguments.

Keeping the Holidays Happy

It's wonderful to be able to celebrate holidays vegan-style, but attending nonvegan holiday gatherings can get complicated. All the food looks extra-good, and your child may feel like the party isn't a party unless he can sample the appetizers and indulge in the sparkly cookies and creamy pies. Investing time to explain to him what he can and cannot eat and why, and making a couple of his favorite vegan dishes and desserts to add to the party table, goes a long way toward making holiday parties a fun experience for everyone.

Holidays are a great time to host a party and introduce family and friends to the best of vegan fare, or to keep it simple and celebrate as a family alone. Our family's favorite holiday meal includes appetizers of vegan polenta with fresh basil and tomato dipping sauce; an olive, fruit, and nut tray; and hummus with black-olive-and-rosemary soft breadsticks. For the main dish, we serve barbecued tofu with cranberry relish. Rounding it out are sides like mashed potatoes, sweet blended buttercup/butternut squash, corn on the cob, and crescent rolls. For dessert? Pumpkin cheesecake.

Kids love it when you incorporate color themes into holiday meals. Here are some ideas to add some color:

♦ For Christmas Eve, serve red sauce pizza and green salad.

♦ For the Fourth of July, go for a veg cookout with red (strawberry), white (vegan cream cheese), and blueberry dessert bars.

♦ And don't forget the bright red box of vegan chocolates on Valentine's Day! (Our favorite is made by Rose City Chocolatiers—www. rosecitychocolates.com.)

> **That's So Vegan**
>
> Find an entire list of vegan Thanksgiving-style recipes at vegweb.com/ index.php?board=304.0. VegWeb.com is one of the most comprehensive veg recipe sites in the world.

Keep your kids in the holiday mix with traditions. Host neighborhood potlucks for other veg or veg-friendly families. Try your hand at veganizing old family favorites. You may be surprised at how close you can come to making Grandma's famous wedding cookies taste exactly like hers but without the dairy or eggs.

And while holidays are a primo opportunity to show off vegan skills, it's also smart to take some of the focus off of food, gifts, and big-money events for your kids and move it toward family time. That way, when they go to the relatives' for a holiday, food won't seem like the end-all, be-all of the event.

Crowd Pleasers

Unless you live in an intentional vegan community, it's pretty safe to say that most of your kids' friends, classmates, and neighbors aren't vegan. So you need a few crowd-pleasing standards for omnivorous kids you feed during play dates, sleepovers, potlucks, parties, and barbecues.

For a quick omni/veg mixed play date or sleepover dinner, meat substitutes are the winner because many of them are barely distinguishable from the animal-based version. Vegan chicken nuggets, chicken patties, or burger crumbles for chili or tacos are great choices. Pair them with some fun-shape pasta served with vegan butter and vegan Parmesan cheese. End with some fruit or Tofutti Cuties for dessert, and you've got yourself a thumbs-up meal! If you want to avoid meat analogs, other good bets are the Tofu Dunkers with dipping sauces (recipe in Chapter 13), A-B-Vegan Soup (recipe in Chapter 13), or any of Amy's Kitchen's brand veg meals. If all else fails, there's always peanut butter and jelly!

Potlucks, parties, and barbecues are fun because most people at parties, including kids, are usually more apt to try new foods, and discussion often centers on tastes, ingredients, and recipes. Our Everything in a Blanket appetizers (recipe later in this chapter) will fly off the trays at your next party. Bring the Barbecue Tofu (recipe later in this chapter), which is easily transportable and tastes good hot, warm, or cold, to your next potluck. Try to bring more than one dish so your kids will have at least a few different veg options, in addition to the usual fruit and veggie trays at most events. Just as with holiday parties, prep your kids beforehand about what they can and cannot eat and what favorites you are bringing for them.

Parent Trap

To avoid any awkward social moments when grilling out is the main event at a party, ask the host if it's okay if you bring your own veggie burgers and veggie dogs to cook on their grill for your family. If you're hosting the cookout, decide ahead of time whether your nonveg guests can cook their own meat on your grill or if you'd prefer it to be all-veg, and let your guests know ahead of time so there are no surprises on either side.

Barbecue Tofu

This barbecue tofu is crispy on the outside and juicy on the inside. You can make it mild or spicy, depending on the sauce you slather on.

$\frac{1}{3}$ cup peanut butter

$\frac{1}{3}$ cup olive oil

1 TB. maple syrup

1 TB. *blackstrap molasses*

1$\frac{1}{2}$ tsp. paprika

1 tsp. salt

$\frac{1}{2}$ tsp. onion powder

$\frac{1}{2}$ tsp. garlic powder

2 (1-lb.) pkg. extra-firm tofu

$\frac{3}{4}$ cup jarred barbecue sauce

Yield: 12 pieces
Prep time: 20 minutes
Cook time: 1 hour, 5 minutes
Serving size: 2 or 3 pieces

1. Preheat the oven to 400°F. Lightly coat a 9×12-inch glass baking dish with nonstick vegetable spray.

2. In a 1-quart bowl, mix together peanut butter, olive oil, maple syrup, blackstrap molasses, paprika, salt, onion powder, and garlic powder with a spoon for 2 or 3 minutes or until smooth.

3. Drain and dry each block of tofu by wrapping it in paper towels and squeezing over the sink. Cut each block into 6 rectangular pieces, for a total of 12 pieces.

4. Place tofu in the prepared baking dish, and using a small spoon, drizzle peanut butter mixture over top of each piece of tofu, spreading it out evenly over each piece. Flip over tofu, and coat other sides.

A B C **Vegan Vocab**

Sticky, slow-running **blackstrap molasses** is derived from sugar cane. Unlike other sugars, it's actually healthy in many regards, adding a sweet source of calcium, magnesium, and potassium, and is especially a great source of iron. From sauces to cookies or beans, this secret ingredient is a sweetly healthy surprise.

5. Bake for 30 minutes. Remove from the oven, flip over tofu using a spatula, and bake for 30 more minutes.

6. Remove from the oven. With a marinade brush, lightly coat each side of tofu pieces with barbecue sauce. Bake for 5 more minutes. Serve directly from the pan or on individual plates with more barbecue sauce and maybe cranberry relish to dip.

Garbanzo Bean–Curry Tofu

Mildly spicy, rich, and creamy, this tofu dish is a weekly standard in our home.

1 (28-oz.) can coconut milk

2 or 3 TB. mild yellow *curry* powder

1 (1-lb.) pkg. extra- or super-firm tofu

$\frac{1}{2}$ cup frozen green peas

1 (14-oz.) can garbanzo beans

2 cups fresh spinach leaves (optional)

$1\frac{1}{2}$ cups dry or 3 cups cooked basmati rice

Yield: 5 cups curry tofu, 3 cups cooked rice

Prep time:
20 minutes

Cook time:
15 minutes

Serving size:
1 cup curry tofu, $\frac{1}{2}$ to $\frac{3}{4}$ cup rice

1. In a large, high-sided cast-iron skillet over medium-low heat, heat coconut milk. Gently swirl in curry powder with a large spoon.

2. Drain and dry block of tofu by wrapping it in paper towels and squeezing over the sink. Cut tofu into 1-inch cubes.

3. Add tofu, frozen peas, and garbanzo beans, and gently blend in to cover with yellow curry. Cook for 10 to 15 minutes. If mixture starts to bubble, reduce heat to low or turn it off.

4. Add spinach (if using) at the last minute, and cook just long enough to wilt it slightly but so it retains its color.

5. Divide cooked rice among individual bowls, ladle curry mixture over top, and serve.

Variation: If adults want to pump up the flavors in this dish, cook the spinach and 1 onion, thinly sliced, in a small frying pan. Mix in 1 teaspoon hot curry powder and a dash of salt. Place curried onion and spinach over rice and tofu curry mixture just for adult servings.

Vegan Vocab

Curry, which is really a catchall term for a combination of traditional Indian spices, may seem too exotic for kids. But in our experience, a mild yellow curry in coconut milk is more palatable to many kids than common American spices such as oregano, black pepper, and parsley.

Everything in a Blanket

This warm, hearty, vegan version of pigs in a blanket is a major leap forward in the concept. Supply dipping sauces of various mustards, ketchup, and other condiments for added flavor.

4 pieces various vegan meat analogs (chik patties, veggie dogs, tempeh bacon, barbecue riblets, veggie burgers, etc.)

1 tube Pillsbury Crescent Rolls

Yield: 8 servings
Prep time: 10 to 15 minutes
Cook time: 11 to 13 minutes
Serving size: 1 sandwich

1. Preheat the oven to 375°F.

2. Cook vegan meat analogs according to package directions. (We use ones that can be microwaved or pan-fried for speediness.) Cut each to fit into 1 crescent roll (usually in half).

3. Unroll crescent rolls onto a baking sheet.

That's So Vegan

These little treats are perfect finger food for party appetizers or sleepovers. Add your own favorite meat substitute products.

4. Place 1 piece cooked vegan meat substitute inside largest end of each crescent roll, and roll up. (Ends of veggie meat will be slightly sticking out sides of rolls.)

5. Bake for 11 to 13 minutes. Serve with your choice of dipping sauces.

Goulash

Belly-warming pasta shells bask in a coating of sweet sauce. Serve with vegan coleslaw and garlic bread.

1 (16-oz.) box medium shell pasta

2 TB. olive oil

$\frac{1}{2}$ cup onion, diced very finely, or 1 tsp. onion powder

1 cup celery, sliced thinly

1 (28-oz.) can tomato purée

$\frac{3}{4}$ cup ketchup

1 tsp. garlic powder

1 tsp. salt

2 tsp. celery salt

1 (15-oz.) can kidney beans, drained and rinsed

2 TB. vegan Parmesan cheese or shredded vegan rice mozzarella (optional)

Yield: 8 cups
Prep time:
30 minutes
Cook time:
20 minutes
Serving size:
1 cup

1. Prepare pasta shells according to package directions. Drain and set aside.

2. In a large, high-sided cast-iron skillet over medium-high heat, heat olive oil. Add onion and celery, and sauté for about 3 minutes, stirring constantly, or until translucent but not browned.

3. Add tomato purée, ketchup, garlic powder, salt, celery salt, and kidney beans, and stir. Cover, reduce heat to low, and simmer for at least 10 minutes or until right before ready to serve.

4. Add cooked pasta, stir, and ladle into shallow bowls. Sprinkle with vegan Parmesan cheese or shredded vegan rice mozzarella (if using).

That's So Vegan

This dish is a good introduction to beans for kids who don't particularly like them because most of the beans in this recipe hide inside the pasta shells! For an adult variation, add in 1 chunked, sautéed green or red pepper, fresh spinach, and ground black pepper or red pepper flakes.

Red Beans

These rich and saucy beans, with their high nutrient value thanks to the puréed onion, garlic, and pepper, make the extra prep time worthwhile.

1 (16-oz.) bag dried small red beans

8 to 10 cups hot water

1 large onion, skins cut off and left whole

1 large green bell pepper, ribs and seeds removed, and cut in $\frac{1}{2}$

6 large cloves garlic, peeled and left whole

$\frac{1}{4}$ cup blackstrap molasses

1 TB. apple cider vinegar

1 TB. Bragg's Liquid Amino Acids

1 tsp. cumin

2 tsp. salt

Yield: 8 to 16 servings

Prep time:
45 minutes

Cook time:
$2\frac{1}{2}$ hours (shorter if you soak beans overnight)

Serving size:
$\frac{1}{2}$ to 1 cup

1. Rinse beans and pick over.

2. In a *Dutch oven* over high heat, combine hot water and beans. (Do not salt water, or beans won't soften.) Bring to a boil, and boil for 2 minutes. Cover and set aside for 1 hour.

3. After 1 hour, add onion, green bell pepper, and garlic cloves to the pan. Onion and pepper should be submerged or just peeking out of water. If not, add more water.

4. Bring to a boil over medium-high heat. Reduce heat to medium-low, and simmer at a slow bubble for 1 to $1\frac{1}{2}$ hours or until beans are tender.

5. With a ladle, remove about 1 cup beans, 1 cup water, onion, bell pepper halves, and 6 garlic cloves from the pan and place in a blender. Purée until smooth and there's no sign of onion, pepper, or garlic cloves. Return purée to rest of beans in the pan.

6. Pour in blackstrap molasses, apple cider vinegar, Bragg's Liquid Amino Acids, and cumin. Simmer at a slow bubble, uncovered, for 15 minutes to 1 hour or until desired thickness.

7. Right before serving, stir in salt. Serve over rice, on tortillas, chips, or alone.

Vegan Vocab _____

A **Dutch oven** is a large cooking pot with thick walls and usually at least 6 quarts in size. With tight-fitting lids and deep sides, Dutch ovens can be made from a number of materials, including cast iron and ceramic, and are perfect for big pots of beans, stews, soups, casseroles, and sauces that can be simmered, enjoyed, and still have plentiful left-overs for freezing and reheating.

Vegan Mashed Potatoes

This is warm, creamy comfort food at its best. Add a bit of vegan sour cream, roasted garlic, garlic powder, or chives for a tasty twist.

6 medium white or yellow potatoes (approx 2 lb.), peeled and quartered

3 TB. vegan butter or margarine, cut into thirds

¼ cup plain soy milk

1 tsp. salt

Yield: 4 servings
Prep time: 15 minutes
Cook time: 35 minutes
Serving size: 1 cup

1. Fill a deep pot with water, and set over high heat. Add potatoes, and bring to a boil. Boil for 20 minutes or until fork-tender. Drain potatoes.

2. Add butter, soy milk, and salt, and mash potatoes with a hand masher for 3 to 5 minutes or until smooth.

3. Stir with a wooden spoon to test consistency. If potatoes are still lumpy or are a bit dry, add more soy milk, 1 tablespoon at a time, and stir.

That's So Vegan

You'll likely find many recipes for vegan gravy, as well as premade vegan gravies in jars and ready-to-make gravy in dry packets, but we have yet to find one we can recommend as kid-friendly. They're either too gel-like or too runny, flavorless, or overly reliant on mushrooms. We don't think you'll miss it on these moist, flavorful potatoes, though. If you want even more creaminess, stir in a couple tablespoons vegan sour cream.

Vegan Home Fries

These thick, chewy home fries will forever change how your kids view fast-food french fries. The salt-free spice coating gives the fries an added kick and a little more crispiness to the outside of the fries.

4 medium to large (at least 5 in. long) baking potatoes

Olive oil–based cooking spray or high-heat sunflower oil cooking spray

1 TB. salt-free table blend seasoning

Yield: 4 servings
Prep time:
10 minutes
Cook time:
20 to 30 minutes
Serving size:
4 to 8 home fries

1. Preheat the oven to 425°F. Coat a baking sheet with cooking spray.

2. Wash and peel potatoes, and cut lengthwise into fourths or eighths. Place onto the prepared baking sheet, and spray potatoes with olive oil–based cooking spray.

3. Sprinkle salt-free table blend seasoning evenly over potatoes.

4. Bake for 10 to 15 minutes, and flip over potatoes with a fork. Cook for 10 to 15 more minutes or until browned and fork-tender. Remove from the oven, and place in a paper towel–lined bowl or basket, and serve.

That's So Vegan

Perfect at the next cookout, with vegan sloppy joes, or as Sunday afternoon football half-time snacks, these home fries are nearly fat-free, which means you and your kids can enjoy them guilt free. Dip in vegan sour cream mixed with chives for an extra-special treat. Or for more spice, turn up the heat with a spicy salt-free seasoning blend.

Chapter 15

Super Snacks

In This Chapter

- ◆ The importance of snacks
- ◆ Easy snacks for vegan kids of all ages
- ◆ Simple yet tasty on-the-go snacks

Throw out that rusty three-meals-a-day rule: vegan kids should be encouraged to snack more often than their omnivorous pals. Growing kids need lots of fuel to fire their active bodies. For many vegan children and teens, a healthful diet based on fruits, vegetables, and whole grains may need a calorie boost. Regularly eating high-calorie, healthy-fat snack foods like nuts and nut butters can mean extra pounds for sedentary adults, but they're just what the doctor ordered for growing vegan kids.

So let's get snacking! The ideas and recipes in this chapter are nutrition-packed and simple to keep close at hand. Whether at home or on the go, your kids need easy access to snack foods that won't melt in pockets or backpacks, don't require refrigeration (thanks to no dairy and eggs), and call out to be devoured.

Why Vegan Kids Need to Snack

According to the American Academy of Pediatrics (AAP), children whose diets are primarily made up of fruits, vegetables, and cereals can develop energy deficits. The high-fiber bulk of these healthful, nutrient-packed foods may cause many children to feel full on fewer *calories* than they need. Long term, that's usually fine—smaller adults tend to be healthier adults. Healthy kids hanging out on the low end of the growth curve may be fine, but falling off the growth curve is not. For active, growing vegan kids, the more healthful food, the better.

Snacking throughout the day boosts kids' caloric intake. Include in their lunch boxes or in the kitchen snack jar naturally fat-rich snack foods like nuts, nut butters, seeds, and certain fruits and veggies like avocadoes and olives. Also, the AAP recommends that parents choose some refined grains rather than all whole grains. Peel some of the fruits and vegetables your child eats. This will cut bulk and promote feelings of hunger, which will make your child likely to eat more.

> **Vegan Vocab**
>
> A **calorie**—or a kilocalorie, as it's more scientifically called—is a measure of the energy value of particular foods.

You don't need to obsessively count every calorie your child eats, but by being aware of the energy value of particular foods, you can choose healthful, calorie-dense snacks for your active child, especially if she isn't gaining weight at an appropriate rate for her age.

Snacks for Toddlers

Not all snacks are created equal, and you need to be age-appropriate with what you serve. With that in mind, here are some easy-to-eat vegan snacks for toddlers:

◆ Bananas, diced to bite size

◆ Small peeled apple slices, diced to bite size

◆ Cheerios

◆ Whole-grain toast with vegan butter

- Vegan graham crackers, including chocolate and cinnamon Teddy Grahams

- Breast milk or soy milk (for toddlers over age 1)

Snacks for Children and Tweens

The keywords here are *self-service.* Most parents wisely want to avoid power struggles over food with their older kids and teens, so set up the environment for healthful snacking success by enticing with color, flavor, and convenience. Present some options, and leave your kids to their own snack choices.

Here are some at-home snack ideas for younger kids:

- Seasonal fruit in an attractive bowl stationed in the middle of the kitchen table

- A well-appointed snack tray in the fridge filled with vegan choices like cut veggies next to Vegan Dill Dip (recipe later in this chapter), Hummus (recipe later in this chapter), or nut butter

- Individual cartons of vegan yogurt with some vegan chocolate chips and blueberries nearby for sprinkling on top

- A baggie with salted baked tofu cubes

- After-School Smoothie Snack (recipe later in this chapter)

A well-stocked pantry and refrigerator will keep most older kids and teens satisfied with snack options. Here are some ideas:

- Tortilla chips and salsa

- Ready-to-eat olives or garbanzo beans

- Homemade Vegan Pretzels (recipe later in this chapter) dipped in hummus or mustard

- Snack bags of snow peas, baby carrots, honey crisp apples, *clementines,* and "cucumber ice-cream cones" (whole cucumbers peeled $3/4$ of the way down with a small bit of peel left at the bottom for easy holding)

Vegan Vocab _____

Clementines are small citrus fruits. Kids often prefer them to oranges, tangerines, or grapefruit because of their small slices, lack of seeds, and extra-sweet flavor. Just one little clementine provides more than 80 percent of the adult RDA of vitamin C.

♦ Cereal with rice or soy milk

♦ A bag of Tings (think vegan Cheetos but with nutritional yeast for a healthful twist)

And be sure to introduce your kids to bars. No, not that kind of bar! We're talking about some of the easiest, ready-to-go, healthful vegan snacks you can buy. These come in dozens of different flavors and are calorie- and nutrient-rich—and it's easy to keep tabs on how many are left in the box or two in your cupboard so you never come up empty handed. Raw versions are even available. At about $1 per bar, one a day per family member can get pricey, but the nutritional benefits these perfectly transportable, kid- and adult-pleasing bars provide can outweigh the price for many busy families.

Packing a Vegan Snack Bag to Go

This throw-in-the-backpack or stash-in-the-car mix has a top-notch blend of carbs, protein, fiber, sweet, salty, crunchy, and chewy—everything kids and teens love. It won't melt, spoil, or leak, but it will disappear faster than you expect!

In small containers or zipper-lock baggies, pack a mixture of the following:

♦ Tings

♦ Raisins

♦ Dried apricots, mangoes, and apples

♦ Cashews

♦ Soy nuts

♦ Pumpkin seeds

If your child doesn't like a particular ingredient in the mix, substitute with another food of similar nutrient makeup—peanuts for cashews, for example.

Most importantly, snacks need to be readily available quick fixes or able to be made when time allows and stored for days at a time. The snack recipes in this chapter are made from simple, available ingredients. Healthful, quick, and fun, most can be made in minutes. The pretzels are the exception, but they can be made in double batches and frozen, if desired. And they're so fun to make that the extra time is worth it for you and your kids!

Homemade Vegan Pretzels

Chewy on the outside and soft on the inside, these salty treats are a hearty snack.

2 or 3 TB. coarse kosher salt

1 (.25-oz.) pkg. active dry yeast

2 TB. plus $\frac{1}{3}$ cup warm water

$\frac{1}{3}$ cup firmly packed brown sugar

5 cups flour, plus more if necessary

Baking soda

Yield: 24 pretzels

Prep time:
1 hour

Cook time:
30 minutes

Serving size:
1 pretzel

1. Preheat the oven to 475°F. Grease 2 cookie sheets with butter or vegan shortening and sprinkle with coarse kosher salt.

2. In a large bowl, dissolve dry yeast in 2 tablespoons warm water. Add remaining $\frac{1}{3}$ cup warm water and brown sugar, and stir well to combine.

3. Knead in flour 1 cup at a time until mixture forms a smooth ball. Add more flour as needed until ball is formed. (Note: Depending on where you live, the current humidity in the air, and other factors, the exact amount of flour will vary.) Remove from bowl and knead on a countertop for 10 more minutes.

4. Divide dough into 24 pieces. Roll out each piece to a 14-inch strand, and twist into a pretzel shape.

5. Fill a large cast-iron skillet a little more than half full with warm water. Add 1 tablespoon baking soda for each 1 cup water used. Place the skillet over medium-high heat, and bring to a simmer.

> **That's So Vegan**
>
> Most kids like pretzels, and this recipe adds brown sugar for a touch of kid-pleasing sweetness. Dip in yellow mustard for extra zing.

6. Using a spatula, lower 1 pretzel into water and cook for 30 seconds. Transfer pretzel to a cookie sheet and sprinkle with coarse salt. Repeat with remaining pretzels.

7. Bake for 8 minutes or until golden brown. Serve immediately, or let cool and store in an airtight container for a day or 2.

Vegan Dill Dip

Creamy, tangy, and dilly, this dill dip tempts kids to eat more veggies simply as transport items for the dip itself!

$\frac{1}{2}$ cup vegan mayonnaise or sandwich spread

1 cup vegan sour cream

1 tsp. salt

$\frac{1}{4}$ cup chopped fresh dill or 1 TB. dried

1 TB. dried onion soup mix (optional)

Yield: 1 $\frac{1}{2}$ cups
Prep time:
8 minutes
Serving size:
2 or 3 tablespoons

1. In a medium bowl, combine mayonnaise, sour cream, salt, dill, and soup mix (if using). Mix well to combine.

2. Serve with crudités, mostly sliced raw veggies, of all kinds.

That's So Vegan

Think outside the box when making crudités for kids. Inventively cutting red bell peppers into zigzag shapes or slicing carrots into tiny matchstick sizes can entice kids to pick one up, dip, and eat.

Easy Vegan Guacamole

This kid-friendly guac goes light on spice, and we add a couple variations to give it a protein or sweetness boost if your child is more likely to dip into guac with either element added.

4 ripe avocados (but not overly ripe)

$\frac{1}{2}$ tsp. cumin

Juice of $\frac{1}{2}$ lime

$\frac{1}{2}$ tsp. salt or to taste

$\frac{1}{4}$ cup frozen yellow corn or petite lima beans (optional)

1 mango, peeled and diced (optional)

Yield: 1½ cups
Prep time: 10 minutes
Serving size: $\frac{1}{2}$ cup

That's So Vegan

Avocados are an excellent source of monounsaturated fats, the kind that lower cholesterol, keep skin and hair supple and shiny, and provide the fat the human body and mind need to thrive.

1. Peel and pit avocados, slice flesh into 1-inch slices, and place in a bowl. Add cumin and lime juice, and mash together with a fork.

2. Add salt, corn (if using), and mango (if using), and mix well.

3. Serve with tortilla chips, in wrap sandwiches, or as a dip for raw veggies.

Deli Roll-Ups

Salty olives and sweet vegan cream cheese roll up inside thin vegan deli slices to make quick, filling, protein-packed snacks.

4 turkey-style vegan tofu deli slices

4 tsp. vegan cream cheese

4 toothpicks

4 pimento-stuffed green olives

Yield: 2 servings
Prep time: 5 minutes
Serving size: 2 roll-ups

1. Arrange deli slices in a single layer on a plate, and spread 1 teaspoon cream cheese on top side of each.

2. Roll up each deli slice onto itself, so cream cheese is on the inside and it makes a tight roll.

3. Seal with a toothpick stuck through center of slice. Place olive through each toothpick, and serve.

That's So Vegan

We crave very few meat-related foods from our omnivorous child-hoods, but items from the deli, especially Italian delis, are among them. Shaved ham and turkey sandwiches, appetizer rolls like these, pepperoni and Italian sausage—these are convenient, versatile, and flavor-packed. And they now come in vegan alternatives. Your family can enjoy all the flavor of deli food as well as the convenience of quick lunch, snacks, or appetizer possibilities, with none of the animal ingredients.

Mini Nachos

These kid-size mini nachos are protein packed and help introduce picky kids to eating a bit of lettuce, olives, or tomato atop a typically kid-friendly item—tortilla chips.

12 tortilla chips (preferably the scoop/ dip-style kind)

$1/4$ cup vegetarian refried beans

1 TB. sliced green or black olives

$1/4$ cup shredded vegan cheddar cheese (rice derived is best)

2 TB. finely shredded iceberg lettuce

1 TB. finely diced tomato

Mild salsa (optional)

Vegan sour cream (optional)

Yield: 2 servings

Prep time:
10 minutes

Cook time:
About 1 minute

Serving size:
6 nachos

1. Arrange tortilla chips in a single layer on a large, microwave-safe plate.

2. Spread about 1 teaspoon refried beans on each chip, and top with 1 olive slice each. Sprinkle each with a few shreds of the vegan cheddar cheese.

3. Microwave on high for 45 seconds to 1 minute or until cheese is melted. Remove from the microwave, and add bits of lettuce and tomato onto each nacho.

4. Serve with mild salsa and vegan sour cream (if using).

That's So Vegan

Keep a can of vegetarian refried beans in your pantry. Spread and dip these protein-packed, convenient, inexpensive, and versatile wonders on everything from tortilla chips and corn and flour tortillas to celery sticks, breadsticks, bagels, and deli slices. Just be sure to get the vegetarian kind, and always ask at restaurants if the refried beans are suitable for vegetarians.

After-School Smoothie Snack

Depending on the type of juice and yogurt you choose—apple, orange, pink grapefruit, pear, and more—the flavors in this smoothie can morph into deliciously infinite combinations.

1¼ cups natural juice (our favorite brand is Naked Juice)

1 banana, peeled and broken into thirds

1 (6-oz.) pkg. soy yogurt or soy-free coconut milk yogurt

Yield: 2 smoothies

Prep time:
4 minutes

Serving size:
1 cup

1. In a blender, combine juice, banana, and soy yogurt. Blend for 1 minute or until smooth.

2. Pour into a glass, and serve with a straw.

That's So Vegan

This smoothie is a good opportunity to try different soy or soy-free nondairy yogurts to see which one your child likes best. The coconut milk version has 30 percent the adult Recommended Daily Allowance of vitamin B_{12} and live and active yogurt cultures.

Chapter 16

Delectable Desserts

In This Chapter

- ◆ Delicious vegan desserts
- ◆ Cool vegan ice creams
- ◆ Yummy vegan cookies and cakes

Vegan desserts are some of the most delicious on the planet, and many tasty, ready-made vegan desserts are available in stores. These are yummy as is, but they're even better when you spruce them up with quick, at-home additions. For days when you're inspired to DIY, we've given you several of our favorite vegan dessert recipes in this chapter—including our family's Vegan Chocolate Birthday Cake!

These Desserts Are *Vegan?*

The most anticipated food group in our family is dessert. Fortunately, vegan desserts have come a long way in recent years, especially vegan frozen treats like ice cream. And most vegan desserts are relatively, if not completely, guilt-free compared to their nonvegan brethren. Even some popular sweets like Oreos and Swedish Fish candies are vegan.

Some of the most kid-friendly vegan desserts are packaged and sold in major grocery stores. If you can't find something in your local store, ask your grocer to stock items from places like the Alternative Baking Company (its line of vegan cookies are incredible); Tofutti brand vegan ice-cream sandwich cookies called Tofutti Cuties; and Temptation's vegan ice cream, which comes in an amazing array of flavors. Trust us, bugging your grocer to stock these vegan specialty foods or bringing a cooler with you to stock up on these desserts the next time you visit the big city is worth it!

Amy's Kitchen brand carries two oh-so-delicious vegan cakes—chocolate and orange—perfect to serve after quick weeknight dinners. Jazz up the chocolate cake with some strawberries and vegan whipped cream. Drizzle the orange cake with a homemade glaze (we give you a recipe later in this chapter) and blueberries, sliced fresh apricots, or raspberries.

Let Them Eat Birthday Cake!

We admit our birthday cake recipe in this chapter is more sweet, moist, and rich than healthful. Hey, it *is* a birthday cake after all! There are other, perhaps healthier, vegan birthday cake recipes you can try. (For example, check out the Vegetarian Resource Group's page on birthday cakes at www.vrg.org/recipes/vegancakes.htm for a chocolate and a vanilla version, as well as an interesting discussion about veganism and birthday cakes.)

A few packaged vegan cake mixes are now sold in well-stocked grocery stores or health food stores. And if you happen to be a city dweller and can afford a splurge, you could order your child's birthday cake from one of the vegan bakeries popping up in many of America's major cities, especially on the East and West Coasts.

Strawberry Malt Shake

What a healthful, yummy alternative to the dairy-heavy traditional straw-berry ice-cream malt! *(Recipe by Hannah Kaminsky.)*

2 cups fresh strawberries (preferably organic), hulled

1 (12-oz.) pkg. firm silken tofu

1 cup vanilla soy milk

2 TB. barley malt syrup

¼ to ⅓ cup agave syrup

Yield: 2 servings
Prep time:
10 minutes
Serving size:
About 2 cups

1. In a blender, combine strawberries and tofu until thoroughly mixed together. Scrape down the sides of the blender, and process once more until completely smooth.

2. With the blender running, add soy milk and barley malt syrup. Add agave to taste, depending on strawberries' sweetness. Stir and serve.

 That's So Vegan

This recipe comes from *VegNews* magazine's online Recipe Club, which delivers recipes directly to your inbox—for free! Check out other recipes by Hannah Kaminsky at bittersweetblog.wordpress. com.

Banana Mango Cream

This sweet mango and banana cream will make you forget all about dairy versions of ice cream.

2 bananas, peeled and cut into small medallions

1 ripe mango, peeled and diced

3 TB. soy, hazelnut, almond, or rice milk

Yield: 3 servings
Prep time:
2 hours, 10 minutes
Serving size:
$^1/_2$ cup

1. Arrange banana medallions on a plate and cover with plastic wrap. Freeze for at least 2 hours or until solid.

2. Remove frozen bananas from the plate with a fork, and place in a blender. Add mango and milk, and pulse to blend for 2 to 4 minutes or until desired consistency is reached. Serve immediately.

Variation: You can omit the mango, reduce the milk to 1 tablespoon, and make a simple banana cream, or keep the milk at 3 tablespoons and add vegan chocolate chips and have a banana chocolate chip cream.

That's So Vegan

If you want a harder, more dairy ice cream–like experience, put the blended cream back in the freezer in the bowls you'll serve it in and allow it to harden for 30 minutes to an hour.

Chocolate-Chip Cookies

These chewy, light vegan cookies are our veganized version of a popular nonvegan chocolate-chip cookie.

¾ cup vegetable shortening

1¼ cups firmly packed brown sugar

2 TB. soy milk

1 TB. vanilla extract

Egg replacer to equal 2 eggs, prepared according to pkg. directions

1¾ cups cake flour

1 tsp. salt

¾ tsp. baking soda

1 cup vegan chocolate chips

1 cup chopped pecans, macadamia nuts, or walnuts (optional)

Yield: 3 dozen cookies
Prep time: 20 minutes
Cook time: 8 to 10 minutes per batch
Serving size: 1 cookie

1. Preheat the oven to 400°F.

2. In a large mixing bowl, combine vegetable shortening, brown sugar, soy milk, and vanilla extract. Using an electric mixer on medium speed, blend for about 2 minutes or until well blended.

3. Stir in prepared egg replacer, scraping the bottom of the bowl to ensure you get all egg replacer into the mixture. Add cake flour, salt, and baking soda, and stir to combine.

4. Fold in chocolate chips and pecans (if using).

5. Drop dough by the tablespoon 2 inches apart onto an ungreased cookie sheet. (Keep cookies small to maintain shape, or they tend to break up.) Bake for 8 to 10 minutes. Do not overbake.

6. Allow cookies to cool on a cooling rack while you repeat with rest of dough.

That's So Vegan

Almost all semisweet chocolate chips are vegan, but check the label for any hidden nonvegan ingredients like nonsoy lecithin.

Ginger-Molasses Cookies

These chewy, lightly sugar-coated cookies are a good source of iron, thanks to the molasses, and they help your kids learn to love ginger.

³⁄₄ cup vegan margarine or shortening

1 cup plus 2 tsp. sugar

Egg replacer equal to 2 eggs, prepared according to pkg. directions

¹⁄₄ cup molasses

1 tsp. cinnamon

1¹⁄₂ tsp. ground ginger

¹⁄₂ tsp. ground cloves

2 tsp. baking soda

2 cups unbleached all-purpose flour

Yield: 2 dozen cookies
Prep time: 20 to 30 minutes
Cook time: 8 to 10 minutes per batch
Serving size: 1 cookie

1. Preheat the oven to 400°F.

2. In a large bowl, and using an electric mixer on medium-high speed, combine margarine and 1 cup sugar for about 2 minutes or until smooth.

3. Add prepared egg replacer, molasses, cinnamon, ginger, cloves, and baking soda. Beat again until well blended.

4. Add flour and *fold* in with a wooden spoon or rubber scraper until combined.

ABC Vegan Vocab

To **fold** means to blend in *gently* using larger, slower, and gentler stirs with a large wooden spoon or rubber scraper. This helps keep baked goods lighter.

5. Place remaining 2 teaspoons sugar in a small bowl.

6. Roll dough into balls about the size of a golf ball and then roll in sugar lightly to coat. Place cookies 2 inches apart on an ungreased cookie sheet. Bake for 8 to 10 minutes.

7. Allow cookies to cool on a cooling rack while you repeat with rest of dough.

Vegan Chocolate Birthday Cake

This vegan birthday cake is velvety-chocolate, rich, and so very decadent.

Egg replacer to equal 2 eggs, prepared according to pkg. directions

1 cup rice milk

$\frac{1}{2}$ cup sunflower oil

3 tsp. vanilla extract

2 cups sugar

1$\frac{3}{4}$ cups unbleached all-purpose flour

$\frac{3}{4}$ plus $\frac{2}{3}$ cup unsweetened cocoa powder

1$\frac{1}{2}$ tsp. baking powder

1$\frac{1}{2}$ tsp. baking soda

1 tsp. salt

1 cup boiling water

1 stick ($\frac{1}{2}$ cup) vegan margarine

3 cups confectioners' sugar

$\frac{1}{3}$ cup soy milk

> **Yield: 1 (9×13-inch) cake, or 2 (9-inch) round cakes**
>
> **Prep time:**
> 30 to 45 minutes
>
> **Cook time:**
> 30 minutes
>
> **Serving size:**
> 1 (4×4-inch) piece

1. Preheat the oven to 400°F. Lightly grease a 9×13-inch cake pan with vegetable shortening or cooking spray. Lightly dust with flour to coat.

2. In a large bowl, combine prepared egg replacer, rice milk, sunflower oil, and 2 teaspoons vanilla extract.

3. In another large bowl, combine sugar, flour, $\frac{3}{4}$ cup cocoa powder, baking powder, baking soda, and salt. Add to egg mixture, and blend with an electric mixer on medium speed for 3 to 5 minutes or until very smooth.

4. Add boiling water, and fold to combine.

5. Pour batter into the prepared baking pan, and bake for 30 minutes. Test for doneness by inserting a toothpick into the center. If the toothpick comes out clean, it's done. Cool cake on a cooling rack.

6. Meanwhile, with an electric mixer on medium speed, blend softened vegan margarine, remaining $^2/_3$ cup cocoa powder, powdered sugar, soy milk, and remaining 1 teaspoon vanilla extract for 3 minutes or until smooth.

Parent Trap

We've only tried one brand of vegan margarine in this cake—Willow Run—so that's what we recommend. Some lesser-quality vegan margarines can taste and blend quite differently, so use Willow Run if you can.

7. When cake is cooled, gently cut away from the sides of the pan, and flip cake onto a cake plate, glass cutting board, or another clean surface. With frosting at room temperature, gently frost top and sides of cake with a frosting knife. Decorate as desired. Depending on the shape of the pan (round or rectangular) cut into triangle or square pieces, and serve with soy or rice ice cream, if desired.

Banana Cake

This moist, banana cake is a kid- and crowd-pleasing dessert alternative to the standard banana bread. It's also a good way to use overripe bananas.

$\frac{1}{2}$ cup vegan margarine, at room temperature

$1\frac{1}{2}$ cups sugar or equivalent sugar alternative

Egg replacer to equal 2 eggs, prepared according to pkg. directions

2 cups cake flour

$\frac{3}{4}$ tsp. baking powder

$\frac{3}{4}$ tsp. baking soda

$\frac{1}{2}$ tsp. salt

$1\frac{1}{4}$ cups overly ripe mashed bananas

$\frac{1}{4}$ cup vegan sour cream

1 tsp. vanilla extract

Yield: 1 (9×13-inch) cake
Prep time: 20 minutes
Cook time: 25 to 35 minutes
Serving size: 1 (4×4-inch) square

1. Preheat the oven to 350°F. Lightly grease a 9×13-inch cake pan with cooking spray or vegetable shortening.

2. In a large bowl, and using an electric mixer on medium speed, beat margarine and sugar for 2 minutes or until smooth. Add egg replacer, and fold in.

3. In another large bowl, sift together cake flour, baking powder, baking soda, and salt.

4. Add wet ingredients to dry ingredients, and stir gently to combine. Fold in bananas, sour cream, and vanilla extract.

That's So Vegan

Thanks to egg replacer, this cake can be vegan and still remain light and fluffy. A powder made of potato starch, tapioca starch flour, and other vegan leavening agents, egg replacer can stand in for both yolks and whites.

5. Pour batter into the prepared pan, and bake for 25 to 35 minutes. Test for doneness by inserting a toothpick into the center. If the toothpick comes out clean, it's done. Top should be golden brown, not overdone. Cool cake in pan on a cooling rack, and serve directly from the pan.

Variation: You can serve this cake plain or drizzled with Orange Cake Glaze (see recipe below) over the top. Or you can use the chocolate frosting recipe from the Vegan Chocolate Birthday Cake (recipe earlier in this chapter), if you're looking for a chocolate-banana flavor.

≈⌒

Orange Cake Glaze

This glaze adds a sweet, homemade taste to any vegan cake. And it's easily adaptable if you're craving a lemon, lime, or even grapefruit glaze.

$\frac{1}{2}$ cup confectioners' sugar

2 TB. pulp-free orange juice, strained

Yield: $\frac{1}{4}$ cup
Prep time: 2 minutes
Serving size: About 1 teaspoon or to taste

1. In a medium bowl, stir together confectioners' sugar and orange juice with a spoon until creamy and no confectioners' sugar bits remain.

2. Drizzle over cake *immediately before serving*. (It will soak in and not look as pretty or taste as good if it's done too early prior to serving.)

Parent Trap

Most sugar in most grocery stores and even health food stores today isn't likely vegan. When using standard sugar or confectioners' sugar, our policy is to go with the BPO. If vegan sugar is available and affordable, we get that. For an in-depth discussion about sugars and veganism, visit www.vegsource.com/jo/qa/qasugar.htm.

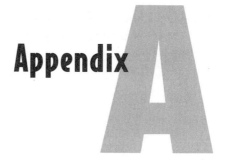

Glossary

best possible option (BPO)   A helpful concept to think about for making the best possible vegan food choice in less-than-ideal situations.

bioavailablity   The amount of a substance, such as a vitamin, the human body can actually use, which can vary depending on many factors, including what other vitamins, minerals, and nutrients are eaten with it.

blackstrap molasses   Sticky, slow-running molasses derived from sugar cane. Unlike other sugars, it's actually healthy in many regards, adding a sweet source of calcium, magnesium, potassium, and is especially a great source of iron.

body mass index (BMI)   A measure of appropriate body size based on weight and height.

calorie   A measure of the energy value of a food.

cholesterol   Is a fat found in all animal fats and oils. It can be found in every cell of the human body and is used to build healthy cells, as well as some vital hormones.

clementine   Small citrus fruits that kids often prefer over oranges, tangerines, or grapefruit because of their small slices, lack of seeds, and extra-sweet flavor. Just one small clementine provides more than 80 percent of the adult RDA of vitamin C.

curry   A catchall term for a combination of traditional Indian spices. It can be mild or spicy to fit children's palates.

docosahexaenoic acid (DHA)   An omega-3 essential fatty acid, important for infant, child, and adult health. Vegans get DHA from algae-sourced supplements and fortified foods.

Dutch oven   A type of large cooking pot with thick walls and usually at least 6 quarts in size; perfect for big pots of beans, stews, soups, casseroles, and sauces.

family medicine doctors   Doctors who complete 3-year residency training programs after medical school, specializing in health care for the whole family. Look for a family medicine physician who is board-certified by the American Board of Family Medicine.

family mission statement   A shared vision of a family's values, plans, and goals as they relate to the current and future functioning of the family—in this case as they relate to veganism.

fold   To gently blend one ingredient into others, not stir or mix, with larger, slower, and gentler stirringlike movements, using a large wooden spoon or rubber scraper. This helps keep baked goods lighter.

heterocyclic amines (HCAs)   Cancer-causing compounds found in cooked meat.

meat analogs   Plant-based foods that closely resemble animal-based counterparts, such as veggie bacon, burgers, sausages, and hot dogs.

nitrites   Preservatives found in cured meats, like hot dogs and pepperoni, that are believed to cause cancers and tumors.

pediatricians   Doctors who complete 3-year residency programs after medical school in caring for children's health needs.

plantains   Fruit that looks like a very large banana that can be fried, mashed, and cooked in many ways, especially when overripe.

satiety   The state of being satisfied or physically full, which is key to lifetime weight management.

standard American diet (SAD)   The sugar- and meat-heavy diet so typical of Westernized populations and quickly spreading throughout the globe. Many health problems, such as obesity, diabetes, certain cancers, and heart disease have been associated with the SAD.

tofu   A product resulting from soybeans that are soaked in water, with a small amount of magnesium chloride, and formed into blocks.

vitamin B_{12}   An important nutrient for red blood cell formation and for healthy nerve tissues. Deficiencies can lead to anemia and permanent nerve and brain damage.

Appendix B

Resources

Kids like to feel part of a community, to connect with other people who experience the world in the same way they do. Many resources are available for vegan kids, and more seem to appear every day. This section provides you with books, websites, movies, and more that can help your child see he's not alone on the vegan road of life.

For you, the parent, find resources on kid-friendly cookbooks, more on child nutrition (some have animal-product sections in them, so just ignore those), and child development/social needs.

Before we mention any other resources for parents, however, we must point to one of the absolute best places to get support on your vegan parent journey: The Vegetarian Resource Group's thousands-strong parent group list. Learn how to sign up at www.vrg.org/family/index.htm.

Kids' Books

Bass, Jules, and Debbie Harter. *Herb, the Vegetarian Dragon*. Cambridge, MA: Barefoot Books, 1999.

Drescher, Henrick. *Hubert the Pudge: A Vegetarian Tale*. Cambridge, MA: Candlewick, 2006.

Newkirk, Ingrid. *50 Awesome Ways Kids Can Help Animals: Fun and Easy Ways to Be a Kind Kid*. New York, NY: Grand Central Publishing, 2006.

Rudy, Sarah. *Benji Bean Sprout Doesn't Eat Meat*. Sacramento, CA: SK Publishing, 2004.

SK Publishing. *Benny Brontosaurus Goes to a Party!* Sacramento, CA: SK Publishing, 2005.

Weiss, Stephanie. *Everything You Need to Know About Being Vegan* (tween/teen book). New York, NY: Rosen Publishing Group, 1999.

Wilder, Laura Ingalls. *The Little House on the Prairie* Series. New York, NY: HarperCollins, 1994.
(These books are not directly vegan, but they do show how farming and the raising and hunting of animals has drastically changed over the generations from the ecological sensitivity and real needs of the Ingalls family to today's ecological degradation, factory farming methods, and hunting for sport.)

Kids' Websites

Humane Society Youth
www.humanesocietyyouth.org

PETA Kids
www.Petakids.com

Roots and Shoots
www.rootsandshoots.org

Kids' Movies

Babe (Universal Studios, 1995)

Charlotte's Web (Paramount, 1973)

Horton Hears a Who! (20th Century Fox, 2008)

Yoga Kids (Gaiam, 2005)

Kid-Friendly Veg Cookbooks

Barnard, Tanya, and Kramer, Sarah. *How It All Vegan*. Vancouver, BC: Arsenal Pulp Press, 1999.

McCann, Jennifer. *Vegan Lunch Box*. Cambridge, MA: Da Capo Press, 2008.

Olson, Cathe. *The Vegetarian Mother's Cookbook*. Arroyo Grande, CA: Goco Publishing, 2005.

Patrick-Goudreau, Colleen. *The Art of Vegan Baking: The Compassionate Cook's Traditional Treats and Sinful Sweets.* Beverly, MA: Fair Winds Press, 2007.

Solomon, Jay. *150 Vegan Favorites.* Roseville, CA: Prima, 1998.

———. *Lean Bean Cuisine.* Roseville, CA: Prima, 1994.

General Child Nutrition

Eisenberg, Arlene, et. al. *What to Expect the First Year.* New York, NY: Workman, 2003.

Pavlina, Erin. *Raising Vegan Children in a Non-Vegan World.* VegFamily.com, 2003.

Sears, William, M.D. *The NDD Book: How Nutrition Deficit Disorder Affects Your Child's Learning, Behavior, and Health, and What You Can Do About It—Without Drugs.* New York, NY: Little, Brown, 2009.

Stepaniak, Joanne, and Vesanto Melina. *Raising Vegetarian Children.* New York, NY: McGraw Hill, 2002.

Ward, Elizabeth. *The Complete Idiot's Guide to Feeding Your Baby and Toddler.* Indianapolis: Alpha Books, 2005.

Child Development/Social Needs

Hartley-Brewer, Elizabeth. *Talking to Tweens: Getting It Right Before It Gets Rocky with Your 8–12-Year-Old.* Cambridge, MA: Da Capo Press, 2005.

Ross, Julie. *How to Hug a Porcupine: Negotiating the Prickly Points of the Tween Years.* New York, NY: McGraw Hill, 2008.

Sears, William, M.D., and Martha Sears, R.N. *The Discipline Book: How to Have a Better Behaved Child from Birth to Age 10.* New York, NY: Little, Brown, 1995.

Weil, Zoe. *Above All, Be Kind: Raising a Humane Child in Challenging Times.* Gabriola Island, BC: New Society Publishers, 2003.

Other Veg Parent Resources

National Co-Op Directory
www.nationalco-opdirectory.com

Nutrition MD
www.nutritionmd.org

**Physicians Committee for
Responsible Medicine**
www.pcrm.org

Raw Families
www.rawfamily.com

**U.S. Centers for Disease Control
BMI Percentile Calculator for
Childs and Teens Age 2 Through 19**
apps.nccd.cdc.gov/dnpabmi

Vegan Families
www.vegfamily.com

Vegan Health
www.veganhealth.org

The Vegan Kitchen
Vegkitchen.com/kid-friendly-recipes.htm

The Vegetarian Resource Group
www.vrg.org

Vegetarian Times
www.vegetariantimes.com

VegNews **Magazine**
www.vegnews.com

Blogs

101 Cookbooks
www.101cookbooks.com

Vegan Blog Tracker
www.vegblogs.com/contact.php

The Post Punk Kitchen
theppk.com/blog

Vegan Lunchbox
veganlunchbox.blogspot.com

VillaVegan
www.villavegan.com

Online Stores

Food Fight Grocery
www.foodfightgrocery.com

KidBean.com
www.kidbean.com

Vegan Essentials
www.veganessentials.com

Vegan Jewelry
www.veganjewelry.com

Index

W–X–Y–Z

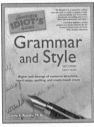
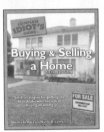
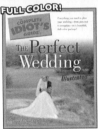
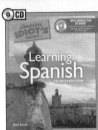
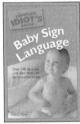
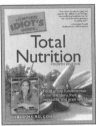
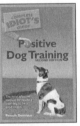
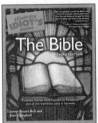
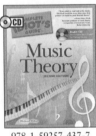
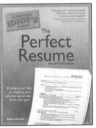
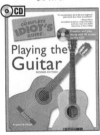
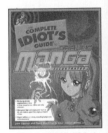
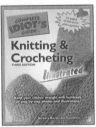
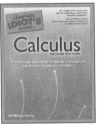
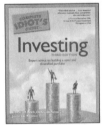